Occupational Ergonomics

Occupational Ergonomics

Edited by
Walter Lennox

Larsen & Keller
www.larsen-keller.com

Occupational Ergonomics
Edited by Walter Lennox
ISBN: 978-1-63549-672-7 (Hardback)

Larsen & Keller
Published by Larsen and Keller Education,
5 Penn Plaza,
19th Floor,
New York, NY 10001, USA

Cataloging-in-Publication Data

Occupational ergonomics / edited by Walter Lennox.
p. cm.
Includes bibliographical references and index.
ISBN 978-1-63549-672-7
1. Human engineering. 2. Industrial engineering. 3. Industrial safety.
4. Industrial hygiene. I. Lennox, Walter.
TA166 .O23 2018
620.82--dc23

Printed and bound in China.

For more information regarding Larsen and Keller Education and its products, please visit the publisher's website www.larsen-keller.com

Table of Contents

Preface

To do efficient work, a person needs to have the proper work environment. Occupational ergonomics refers to the study and practice of providing people with the best-required work environment to boost their work and make it more efficient and optimum. It also includes promoting safety, health and comfort. This book is compiled in such a manner, that it will provide in-depth knowledge about the theory and practice of occupational ergonomics. While understanding the long-term perspectives of the topics, it makes an effort in highlighting their impact as a modern tool for the growth of the discipline. This textbook is an essential guide for both academicians and those who wish to pursue this discipline further.

A short introduction to every chapter is written below to provide an overview of the content of the book:

Chapter 1 - Ergonomics is the study and design of equipments that are used by humans. The emphasis of ergonomics is to provide well-being and comfort to the user. The subject overlaps with numerous disciplines like engineering, industrial design, physiology and biomechanics. The chapter on ergonomics offers an insightful focus, keeping in mind the complex subject matter; **Chapter 2** - Cognitive ergonomics studies mental processes like memory, perception and motor response. It studies human strategies devised as a response to a work process. The significant themes related to the subject matter are decision-making, work stress, workload, skilled performance and human reliability. The chapter serves as a source to understand cognitive ergonomics; **Chapter 3** - Occupational hazards are threats faced by workers in their workplace. It includes hazards such as biological hazards, psychosocial hazards, chemical hazards and physical hazards. The chapter strategically encompasses and incorporates the major components and key concepts of occupational hazards and safety, providing a complete understanding; **Chapter 4** - Occupational diseases are diseases that occur in humans because of their occupational activity. Some examples of known occupational diseases are lung diseases, skin diseases, etc. Occupational injuries are injuries sustained in the workplace, especially while carrying out hazardous work. The topics elaborated in this chapter will help in gaining a better perspective about physical ergonomics; **Chapter 5** - The diverse aspects of occupational ergonomics are Rohmert's law, engineering psychology, workplace aggression, etc. Any type of aggression which occurs in the workplace is known as workplace aggression. The behavior ranges from verbal abuses to degrading a person to physical abuse. This chapter has been carefully written to provide an easy understanding of the diverse aspects of occupational ergonomics.

I extend my sincere thanks to the publisher for considering me worthy of this task. Finally, I thank my family for being a source of support and help.

Editor

1

An Overview of Ergonomics

Ergonomics is the study and design of equipments that are used by humans. The emphasis of ergonomics is to provide well-being and comfort to the user. The subject overlaps with numerous disciplines like engineering, industrial design, physiology and biomechanics. The chapter on ergonomics offers an insightful focus, keeping in mind the complex subject matter.

Human Factors and Ergonomics

Human factors and ergonomics (commonly referred to as HF&E), also known as comfort design, functional design, and systems, is the practice of designing products, systems, or processes to take proper account of the interaction between them and the people who use them.

The field has seen some contributions from numerous disciplines, such as psychology, engineering, biomechanics, industrial design, physiology, and anthropometry. In essence, it is the study of designing equipment, devices and processes that fit the human body and its cognitive abilities. The two terms "human factors" and "ergonomics" are essentially synonymous.

The International Ergonomics Association defines ergonomics or human factors as follows:

Ergonomics (or human factors) is the scientific discipline concerned with the understanding of interactions among humans and other elements of a system, and the profession that applies theory, principles, data and methods to design in order to optimize human well-being and overall system performance.

HF&E is employed to fulfill the goals of occupational health and safety and productivity. It is relevant in the design of such things as safe furniture and easy-to-use interfaces to machines and equipment.

Proper ergonomic design is necessary to prevent repetitive strain injuries and other musculoskeletal disorders, which can develop over time and can lead to long-term disability.

Human factors and ergonomics is concerned with the "fit" between the user, equipment and their environments. It takes account of the user's capabilities and limitations in seeking to ensure that tasks, functions, information and the environment suit each user.

To assess the fit between a person and the used technology, human factors specialists or ergonomists consider the job (activity) being done and the demands on the user; the equipment used (its size, shape, and how appropriate it is for the task), and the information used (how it is presented, accessed, and changed). Ergonomics draws on many disciplines in its study of humans and their environments, including anthropometry, biomechanics, mechanical engineering, industrial engineering, industrial design, information design, kinesiology, physiology, cognitive psychology, industrial and organizational psychology, and space psychology.

Etymology

The term *ergonomics* first entered the modern lexicon when Polish scientist Wojciech Jastrzębowski used the word in his 1857 article *Rys ergonomji czyli nauki o pracy, opartej na prawdach poczerpniętych z Nauki Przyrody* (The Outline of Ergonomics; i.e. Science of Work, Based on the Truths Taken from the Natural Science). The introduction of the term to the English lexicon is widely attributed to British psychologist Hywel Murrell, at the 1949 meeting at the UK's Admiralty, which led to the foundation of The Ergonomics Society. He used it to encompass the studies in which he had been engaged during and after World War II.

The expression *human factors* is a predominantly North American term which has been adopted to emphasise the application of the same methods to non work-related situations. A "human factor" is a physical or cognitive property of an individual or social behavior specific to humans that may influence the functioning of technological systems. The terms "human factors" and "ergonomics" are essentially synonymous.

Domains of Specialization

Ergonomics comprise three main fields of research: Physical, cognitive and organisational ergonomics.

There are many specializations within these broad categories. Specialisations in the field of physical ergonomics may include visual ergonomics. Specialisations within the field of cognitive ergonomics may include usability, human–computer interaction, and user experience engineering.

Some specialisations may cut across these domains: *Environmental ergonomics* is concerned with human interaction with the environment as characterized by climate, temperature, pressure, vibration, light. The emerging field of human factors in highway safety uses human factor principles to understand the actions and capabilities of road users – car and truck drivers, pedestrians, bicyclists, etc. – and use this knowledge to design roads and streets to reduce traffic collisions. Driver error is listed as a contributing factor in 44% of fatal collisions in the United States, so a topic of particular interest is how road users gather and process information about the road and its environment, and how to assist them to make the appropriate decision.

New terms are being generated all the time. For instance, "user trial engineer" may refer to a human factors professional who specialises in user trials. Although the names change, human factors professionals apply an understanding of human factors to the design of equipment, systems and working methods in order to improve comfort, health, safety, and productivity.

According to the International Ergonomics Association, within the discipline of ergonomics there exist domains of specialization:

Physical Ergonomics

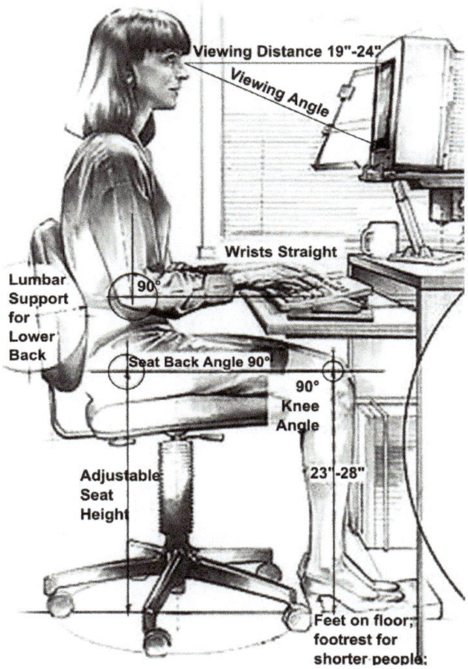

Physical ergonomics: the science of designing user interaction with equipment and workplaces to fit the user.

Physical ergonomics is concerned with human anatomy, and some of the anthropometric, physiological and bio mechanical characteristics as they relate to physical activity. Physical ergonomic principles have been widely used in the design of both consumer and industrial products. Physical ergonomics is important in the medical field, particularly to those diagnosed with physiological ailments or disorders such as arthritis (both chronic and temporary) or carpal tunnel syndrome. Pressure that is insignificant or imperceptible to those unaffected by these disorders may be very painful, or render a device unusable, for those who are. Many ergonomically designed products are also used or recommended to treat or prevent such disorders, and to treat pressure-related chronic pain.

One of the most prevalent types of work-related injuries is musculoskeletal disorder. Work-related musculoskeletal disorders (WRMDs) result in persistent pain, loss of functional capacity and work disability, but their initial diagnosis is difficult because they are mainly based on complaints of pain and other symptoms. Every year, 1.8 million U.S. workers experience WRMDs and nearly 600,000 of the injuries are serious enough to cause workers to miss work. Certain jobs or work conditions cause a higher rate of worker complaints of undue strain, localized fatigue, discomfort, or pain that does not go away after overnight rest. These types of jobs are often those involving activities such as repetitive and forceful exertions; frequent, heavy, or overhead lifts; awkward work positions; or use of vibrating equipment. The Occupational Safety and Health Administration (OSHA) has found substantial evidence that ergonomics programs can cut workers' compensation costs, increase productivity and decrease employee turnover. Therefore, it is important to gather data to identify jobs or work conditions that are most problematic, using sources such as injury and illness logs, medical records, and job analyses.

Cognitive Ergonomics

Cognitive ergonomics is concerned with mental processes, such as perception, memory, reasoning, and motor response, as they affect interactions among humans and other elements of a system. (Relevant topics include mental workload, decision-making, skilled performance, human reliability, work stress and training as these may relate to human-system and Human-Computer Interaction design.)

Organizational Ergonomics

Organizational ergonomics is concerned with the optimization of socio-technical systems, including their organizational structures, policies, and processes. (Relevant topics include communication, crew resource management, work design, work systems, design of working times, teamwork, participatory design, community ergonomics, cooperative work, new work programs, virtual organizations, telework, and quality management.)

History of the Field

In Ancient Societies

The foundations of the science of ergonomics appear to have been laid within the context of the culture of Ancient Greece. A good deal of evidence indicates that Greek civilization in the 5th century BC used ergonomic principles in the design of their tools, jobs, and workplaces. One outstanding example of this can be found in the description Hippocrates gave of how a surgeon's workplace should be designed and how the tools he uses should be arranged. The archaeological record also shows that the early Egyptian dynasties made tools and household equipment that illustrated ergonomic principles.

In Industrial Societies

In the 19th century, Frederick Winslow Taylor pioneered the "scientific management" method, which proposed a way to find the optimum method of carrying out a given task. Taylor found that he could, for example, triple the amount of coal that workers were shoveling by incrementally reducing the size and weight of coal shovels until the fastest shoveling rate was reached. Frank and Lillian Gilbreth expanded Taylor's methods in the early 1900s to develop the "time and motion study". They aimed to improve efficiency by eliminating unnecessary steps and actions. By applying this approach, the Gilbreths reduced the number of motions in bricklaying from 18 to 4.5, allowing bricklayers to increase their productivity from 120 to 350 bricks per hour.

However, this approach was rejected by Russian researchers who focused on the well being of the worker. At the First Conference on Scientific Organization of Labour (1921) Vladimir Bekhterev and Vladimir Nikolayevich Myasishchev criticised Taylorism. Bekhterev argued that "The ultimate ideal of the labour problem is not in it [Taylorism], but is in such organisation of the labour process that would yield a maximum of efficiency coupled with a minimum of health hazards, absence of fatigue and a guarantee of the sound health and all round personal development of the working people." Myasishchev rejected Frederick Taylor's proposal to turn man into a machine. Dull monotonous work was a temporary necessity until a corresponding machine can be developed. He also went on to suggest a new discipline of "ergology" to study work as an integral part of the re-organisation of work. The concept was taken up by Myasishchev's mentor, Bekhterev, in his final report on the conference, merely changing the name to "ergonology"

In Aviation

Prior to World War I, the focus of aviation psychology was on the aviator himself, but the war shifted the focus onto the aircraft, in particular, the design of controls and displays, and the effects of altitude and environmental factors on the pilot. The war saw the emergence of aeromedical research and the need for testing and measurement methods. Studies on driver behaviour started gaining momentum during this period, as Henry Ford started providing millions of Americans with automobiles. Another major development during this period was the performance of aeromedical research. By the end of World War I, two aeronautical labs were established, one at Brooks Air Force Base, Texas and the other at Wright-Patterson Air Force Base outside of Dayton, Ohio. Many tests were conducted to determine which characteristic differentiated the successful pilots from the unsuccessful ones. During the early 1930s, Edwin Link developed the first flight simulator. The trend continued and more sophisticated simulators and test equipment were developed. Another significant development was in the civilian sector, where the effects of illumination on worker productivity were examined. This led to the identification of the Hawthorne Effect, which suggested that motivational factors could significantly influence human performance.

World War II marked the development of new and complex machines and weaponry, and these made new demands on operators' cognition. It was no longer possible to adopt the Tayloristic principle of matching individuals to preexisting jobs. Now the design of equipment had to take into account human limitations and take advantage of human capabilities. The decision-making, attention, situational awareness and hand-eye coordination of the machine's operator became key in the success or failure of a task. There was substantial research conducted to determine the human capabilities and limitations that had to be accomplished. A lot of this research took off where the aeromedical research between the wars had left off. An example of this is the study done by Fitts and Jones (1947), who studied the most effective configuration of control knobs to be used in aircraft cockpits.

Much of this research transcended into other equipment with the aim of making the controls and displays easier for the operators to use. The entry of the terms "human factors" and "ergonomics" into the modern lexicon date from this period. It was observed that fully functional aircraft flown by the best-trained pilots, still crashed. In 1943 Alphonse Chapanis, a lieutenant in the U.S. Army, showed that this so-called "pilot error" could be greatly reduced when more logical and differentiable controls replaced confusing designs in airplane cockpits. After the war, the Army Air Force published 19 volumes summarizing what had been established from research during the war.

In the decades since World War II, HF&E has continued to flourish and diversify. Work by Elias Porter and others within the RAND Corporation after WWII extended the conception of HF&E. "As the thinking progressed, a new concept developed—that it was possible to view an organization such as an air-defense, man-machine system as a single organism and that it was possible to study the behavior of such an organism. It was the climate for a breakthrough." In the initial 20 years after the World War II, most activities were done by the "founding fathers": Alphonse Chapanis, Paul Fitts, and Small.

During the Cold War

The beginning of the Cold War led to a major expansion of Defense supported research laboratories. Also, many labs established during WWII started expanding. Most of the research following the war was military-sponsored. Large sums of money were granted to universities to conduct research. The scope of the research also broadened from small equipments to entire workstations and systems. Concurrently, a lot of opportunities started opening up in the civilian industry. The focus shifted from research to participation through advice to engineers in the design of equipment. After 1965, the period saw a maturation of the discipline. The field has expanded with the development of the computer and computer applications.

The Space Age created new human factors issues such as weightlessness and extreme g-forces. Tolerance of the harsh environment of space and its effects on the mind and body were widely studied

Information Age

The dawn of the Information Age has resulted in the related field of human–computer interaction (HCI). Likewise, the growing demand for and competition among consumer goods and electronics has resulted in more companies and industries including human factors in their product design. Using advanced technologies in human kinetics, body-mapping, movement patterns and heat zones, companies are able to manufacture purpose-specific garments, including full body suits, jerseys, shorts, shoes, and even underwear.

In the context of modern footwear ergonomics, the balance of needs between the footwear's ability to conform to the gait of the wearer whilst also providing protection and grip for their feet, is investigated by the use of motion analysis systems, force measurement plates, and in-shoe pressure measurements. The most useful information is obtained when the various factors can be observed simultaneously i.e. foot and leg motion observed and considered in conjunction with in-shoe pressure.

HF&E Organizations

Formed in 1946 in the UK, the oldest professional body for human factors specialists and ergonomists is The Chartered Institute of Ergonomics and Human Factors, formally known as the *Institute of Ergonomics and Human Factors* and before that, *The Ergonomics Society*.

The Human Factors and Ergonomics Society (HFES) was founded in 1957. The Society's mission is to promote the discovery and exchange of knowledge concerning the characteristics of human beings that are applicable to the design of systems and devices of all kinds.

The International Ergonomics Association (IEA) is a federation of ergonomics and human factors societies from around the world. The mission of the IEA is to elaborate and advance ergonomics science and practice, and to improve the quality of life by expanding its scope of application and contribution to society. As of September 2008, the International Ergonomics Association has 46 federated societies and 2 affiliated societies.

Related Organizations

The Institute of Occupational Medicine (IOM) was founded by the coal industry in 1969. From the outset the IOM employed an ergonomics staff to apply ergonomics principles to the design of mining machinery and environments. To this day, the IOM continues ergonomics activities, especially in the fields of musculoskeletal disorders; heat stress and the ergonomics of personal protective equipment (PPE). Like many in occupational ergonomics, the demands and requirements of an ageing UK workforce are a growing concern and interest to IOM ergonomists.

The International Society of Automotive Engineers (SAE) is a professional organization for mobility engineering professionals in the aerospace, automotive, and commercial vehicle industries. The Society is a standards development organization for the engineering of powered vehicles of all kinds, including cars, trucks, boats, aircraft, and others. The Society of Automotive Engineers has established a number of standards used in the automotive industry and elsewhere. It encourages the design of vehicles in accordance with established Human Factors principles. It is one of the most influential organizations with respect to Ergonomics work in Automotive design. This society regularly holds conferences which address topics spanning all aspects of Human Factors/ Ergonomics.

Practitioners

Human factors practitioners come from a variety of backgrounds, though predominantly they are psychologists (from the various subfields of industrial and organizational psychology, engineering psychology, cognitive psychology, perceptual psychology, applied psychology, and experimental psychology) and physiologists. Designers (industrial, interaction, and graphic), anthropologists, technical communication scholars and computer scientists also contribute. Typically, an ergonomist will have an undergraduate degree in psychology, engineering, design or health sciences, and usually a masters degree or doctoral degree in a related discipline. Though some practitioners enter the field of human factors from other disciplines, both M.S. and PhD degrees in Human Factors Engineering are available from several universities worldwide.

Methods

Until recently, methods used to evaluate human factors and ergonomics ranged from simple questionnaires to more complex and expensive usability labs. Some of the more common HF&E methods are listed below:

- Ethnographic analysis: Using methods derived from ethnography, this process focuses on observing the uses of technology in a practical environment. It is a qualitative and observational method that focuses on "real-world" experience and pressures, and the usage of technology or environments in the workplace. The process is best used early in the design process.
- Focus Groups are another form of qualitative research in which one individual will facilitate discussion and elicit opinions about the technology or process under investigation. This can be on a one-to-one interview basis, or in a group session. Can be used to gain a large quantity of deep qualitative data, though due to the small sample size, can be subject to a higher degree of individual bias. Can be used at any point in the design process, as it is largely dependent on the exact questions to be pursued, and the structure of the group. Can be extremely costly.

- Iterative design: Also known as prototyping, the iterative design process seeks to involve users at several stages of design, in order to correct problems as they emerge. As prototypes emerge from the design process, these are subjected to other forms of analysis as outlined in this article, and the results are then taken and incorporated into the new design. Trends amongst users are analyzed, and products redesigned. This can become a costly process, and needs to be done as soon as possible in the design process before designs become too concrete.
- Meta-analysis: A supplementary technique used to examine a wide body of already existing data or literature in order to derive trends or form hypotheses in order to aid design decisions. As part of a literature survey, a meta-analysis can be performed in order to discern a collective trend from individual variables.
- Subjects-in-tandem: Two subjects are asked to work concurrently on a series of tasks while vocalizing their analytical observations. The technique is also known as "Co-Discovery" as participants tend to feed off of each other's comments to generate a richer set of observations than is often possible with the participants separately. This is observed by the researcher, and can be used to discover usability difficulties. This process is usually recorded.
- Surveys and Questionnaires: A commonly used technique outside of Human Factors as well, surveys and questionnaires have an advantage in that they can be administered to a large group of people for relatively low cost, enabling the researcher to gain a large amount of data. The validity of the data obtained is, however, always in question, as the questions must be written and interpreted correctly, and are, by definition, subjective. Those who actually respond are in effect self-selecting as well, widening the gap between the sample and the population further.
- Task analysis: A process with roots in activity theory, task analysis is a way of systematically describing human interaction with a system or process to understand how to match the demands of the system or process to human capabilities. The complexity of this process is generally proportional to the complexity of the task being analyzed, and so can vary in cost and time involvement. It is a qualitative and observational process. Best used early in the design process.
- Think aloud protocol: Also known as "concurrent verbal protocol", this is the process of asking a user to execute a series of tasks or use technology, while continuously verbalizing their thoughts so that a researcher can gain insights as to the users' analytical process. Can be useful for finding design flaws that do not affect task performance, but may have a negative cognitive affect on the user. Also useful for utilizing experts in order to better understand procedural knowledge of the task in question. Less expensive than focus groups, but tends to be more specific and subjective.

- User analysis: This process is based around designing for the attributes of the intended user or operator, establishing the characteristics that define them, creating a persona for the user. Best done at the outset of the design process, a user analysis will attempt to predict the most common users, and the characteristics that they would be assumed to have in common. This can be problematic if the design concept does not match the actual user, or if the identified are too vague to make clear design decisions from. This process is, however, usually quite inexpensive, and commonly used.
- "Wizard of Oz": This is a comparatively uncommon technique but has seen some use in mobile devices. Based upon the Wizard of Oz experiment, this technique involves an operator who remotely controls the operation of a device in order to imitate the response of an actual computer program. It has the advantage of producing a highly changeable set of reactions, but can be quite costly and difficult to undertake.
- Methods Analysis is the process of studying the tasks a worker completes using a step-by-step investigation. Each task in broken down into smaller steps until each motion the worker performs is described. Doing so enables you to see exactly where repetitive or straining tasks occur.
- Time studies determine the time required for a worker to complete each task. Time studies are often used to analyze cyclical jobs. They are considered "event based" studies because time measurements are triggered by the occurrence of predetermined events.
- Work sampling is a method in which the job is sampled at random intervals to determine the proportion of total time spent on a particular task. It provides insight into how often workers are performing tasks which might cause strain on their bodies.
- Predetermined time systems are methods for analyzing the time spent by workers on a particular task. One of the most widely used predetermined time system is called Methods-Time-Measurement (MTM). Other common work measurement systems include MODAPTS and MOST. Industry specific applications based on PTS are Seweasy,MODAPTS and GSD as seen in paper: Miller, Doug, Towards Sustainable Labour Costing in UK Fashion Retail (February 5, 2013).
- Cognitive Walkthrough: This method is a usability inspection method in which the evaluators can apply user perspective to task scenarios to identify design problems. As applied to macroergonomics, evaluators are able to analyze the usability of work system designs to identify how well a work system is organized and how well the workflow is integrated.

- Kansei Method: This is a method that transforms consumer's responses to new products into design specifications. As applied to macroergonomics, this method can translate employee's responses to changes to a work system into design specifications.

- High Integration of Technology, Organization, and People (HITOP): This is a manual procedure done step-by-step to apply technological change to the workplace. It allows managers to be more aware of the human and organizational aspects of their technology plans, allowing them to efficiently integrate technology in these contexts.

- Top Modeler: This model helps manufacturing companies identify the organizational changes needed when new technologies are being considered for their process.

- Computer-integrated Manufacturing, Organization, and People System Design (CIMOP): This model allows for evaluating computer-integrated manufacturing, organization, and people system design based on knowledge of the system.

- Anthropotechnology: This method considers analysis and design modification of systems for the efficient transfer of technology from one culture to another.

- Systems Analysis Tool (SAT): This is a method to conduct systematic trade-off evaluations of work-system intervention alternatives.

- Macroergonomic Analysis of Structure (MAS): This method analyzes the structure of work systems according to their compatibility with unique sociotechnical aspects.

- Macroergonomic Analysis and Design (MEAD): This method assesses work-system processes by using a ten-step process.

- Virtual Manufacturing and Response Surface Methodology (VMRSM): This method uses computerized tools and statistical analysis for workstation design.

Weaknesses

Problems related to measures of usability include the fact that measures of learning and retention of how to use an interface are rarely employed and some studies treat measures of how users interact with interfaces as synonymous with quality-in-use, despite an unclear relation.

Although field methods can be extremely useful because they are conducted in the users' natural environment, they have some major limitations to consider. The limitations include:

1. Usually take more time and resources than other methods
2. Very high effort in planning, recruiting, and executing compared with other methods
3. Much longer study periods and therefore requires much goodwill among the participants
4. Studies are longitudinal in nature, therefore, attrition can become a problem.

Light Ergonomics

Light ergonomics is the relationship between the light source and the individual. Poor light can be divided into the following:

- Individual or socio-cultural expectations
- Insufficient light
- Poor distribution of light
- Improper contrast
- Glare
- Flicker
- Thermal heating (over or under)
- Acoustic noise (especially fluorescents)
- Color spectrum (amber street lighting)

Effects of Poor Light

The effects of poor light can include the following:

- low productivity
- high human error rates
- inability to match or select correct colors
- eyestrain
- headache
- a reduction in mental alertness
- general malaise
- low employee morale

Recommended Illumination Levels	
Type of Activity	**Ranges of Illuminations (Lux)**
Public spaces with dark surroundings	30
Simple orientation for short temporary visits	50
Working spaces where visual tasks are only occasionally performed	100
Performance of visual tasks of high contrast or large scale	300
Performance of visual tasks of medium contrast or small size	500
Performance of visual tasks of low contrast or very small size	1000
Performance of visual tasks near threshold of person's ability to recognize an image	3000-10000

Types of Light Sources

Light Bulbs				
Type	**Common Application**	**Efficiency**	**Colour Rendering**	**Fog-Smog Penetration**
Incandescent	Homes	Poor	Good	
Fluorescent	Home&Office	Good	Fair to good	
Mercury	Factories, offices	Fair	Fair to moderate	
Low pressure sodium	Roadway	Good	Poor	Good
High pressure sodium	Factories, commercial	Good	Fair to good	Good
Metal Halide	Factories, commercial	Good	Good	
Light-emitting diode (LED)	Home & office, commercial, industrial	Excellent	Good	

Human Factors Integration

Human Factors Integration (HFI) is the process adopted by a number of key industries (notably defence and hazardous industries like oil & gas) in Europe to integrate human factors and ergonomics into the systems engineering process. Although each industry has a slightly different domain the underlying approach is the same.

Overview

In essence tries to reconcile the top down nature of system engineering with the iterative nature of a user centred design approach (e.g. ISO 6385 or ISO 9241-210). It often does this by creating a Human Factors Integration Plan (HFIP) that sits alongside the system development plan. The purpose of the HFIP is to define how the Human Factors Engineering activities necessary for the successful delivery of a particular system will be conducted.

It establishes the guiding principles to be followed by the project to implement the best-practice Human Factors methods. As well as the principles involved, the Plan normally describes the organisation, processes and controls necessary over the entire life cycle of the system from the concept phase through to decommissioning.

Domains

HFI undertakes this by conducting a formal process that identifies and reconciles human related issues. These issues are split for convenience into domains. The seven domains defined by the US Army under its MANPRINT programme are:

Manpower - The number of military and civilian personnel required and potentially available to operate, maintain, sustain and provide training for systems

Personnel - The cognitive and physical capabilities required to be able to train for, operate, maintain and sustain systems.

Training - The instruction or education, and on-the-job or unit training required to provide personnel their essential job skills, knowledge, values and attributes.

Human Factors Engineering - The integration of human characteristics into system definition, design, development, and evaluation to optimise human-machine performance under operational conditions.

Health Hazard Assessment - Short or long term hazards to health occurring as a result of normal operation of the system.

System safety - Safety risks occurring when the system is functioning in an abnormal manner.

Soldier Survivability - The characteristics of a system that can reduce fratricide, detectability and probability of being attacked and minimize system damage, soldier injury and cognitive and physical fatigue.

The UK Ministry of Defence (MoD) adopted a similar HFI approach to MANPRINT in the early 1990s, but excluded Soldier Survivability. Subsequently the MoD added a seventh 'Social & Organisational' domain. Some industries also include habitability as a separate domain.

HFI Plan

The HFI plan scope defines the relationship between all the activities and the Human Factors domains and provides a systematic approach to ensure that:

- The human role in the system is defined to optimise human performance in relation to the core system architecture and ancillary equipment.

- Adequate human-equipment analyses and trade-off studies are performed, revisiting the assumptions throughout the system life cycle. The process is iterative. As the programme progresses, the HF activities involve greater depth of analysis.
- Biomedical analysis and design support includes the environmental protection necessary to promote health and safety, and the capability for safe operation and maintenance of the core architecture and ancillary equipment.
- Training characteristics (materials, environment, evaluation criteria, etc.) for system personnel are identified.
- System testing and evaluation is conducted to verify that users can safely and effectively operate, maintain and support equipment in its intended environment.
- The design meets agreed operational performance standards and where this is not the case, to modify the design or associated training in such a way that the resultant manned system meets the required standards.

Activity-centered Ergonomics

Following Maurice de Montmollin (*philosopher and psychologist at the Sorbonne*), the French distinguished generally two major trends in ergonomics:

- Ergonomics focuses on the activity, which emphasizes understanding the work situation as a whole, the demand analysis and framework intervention and the distinction between prescribed work and real work. This school is mainly present in the Francophone countries, Brazil and another form in Scandinavia.
- The ergonomics of the human factors, focusing on research results General (on the postures, rhythms, moods of work ...) and definition of standards. It is dominant in the United States and Japan.

Definitions

Activity-centered ergonomics uses knowledge from the physiology of labor, cognitive psychology (memory attention, collection learning ...) and the psycho-physiology (alert, posture, working conditions ...), sociology of organizations (distribution of functions, organizations in the chain of command, the string functional, social psychology, linguistics, among others: in fact all sciences relating to man).

It is based on models of the work situation (especially that of Jacques Christol, Jacques Leplat and Gilbert De Terssac) that focus on the difference *'nature'* between the task (project record, the field of virtual future) and activity (body – the brain of course) who takes positions and makes movements activates the controls, manages (consciously or not) thought processes, communicate with others, organizes his actions, etc..

The first feature of the analysis of this activity is that the operator "regulates" the activity, according to its external environment, its internal state (e.g. fatigue) to ensure maximum consistency of performance: accelerating the pace of work to catch up with the delay or face an emergency change procedure against poor results ...

The second dominant feature is the concept of compromise between the requirements of performance (explicitly or implicitly always present) and requirements related to compliance with the rules (Security of management, technical, administrative ...). The Observer of the work activity notes*'always'* that this compromise exists, and it is not built as would the organizations, focusing on the rule prescribed first. The reality is complex, as in everyday life, where we all respect the speed limit on the road ... unless we're afraid of missing our train, or arrive late to an urgent appointment ...

This "cognitive compromise" is also affected by aspects psychic s of activity, insofar as studies of psychological aspects of work, increasing show that the achievement of production requires more and more not only to compromise with the security (which is never written) but also with its afraid, its stress his emotions etc.. This compromise can be considered "room", without going on the field with operators in business, whether to make a machine, a workstation or a computer interface: the standards and rules are inadequate ever.

Ergonomics Analysis of Work

Ergonomic analysis of work (EAW) is the main tool of the activity-centered ergonomic intervention. It can help to solve several problems related to working conditions or the design of tools and equipment.

- Aspects of health in work
    - On the physical health including the musculoskeletal disorder (MSD) affecting 12 to 14% of employees
    - On the mental health risks due to particular psycho-social (in stress) can cause anxiety-depressive syndromes (about 8% of employees)
- Aspects of performance
    - Improving productivity
    - Improving quality

EAW, an Influenced Analysis

EAW, a "Located" Analysis

It is with the demand analysis and hypothesis he has made during the pre-diagnosis that the ergonomist will be able to choose situations to consider:

- Ensure sufficient mastery of technical data concerning the work situation;
- Build reference tools for description and interpretation of data;
- Give himself a medium for demonstration and communication.

The Different Elements of Influence on Work

The work activity is influenced by a multitude of facets. The ergonomist must rely on these aspects and compare the actual work for generating insights relevant to the problems posed

- The technical process : These are views which focus on flows and processing steps of a product or information
- The tools and media : An analysis of the means available to employees to obtain or receive information and act on the process to better prepare some investigations
- The relationship between the variables of a device : In explanation with the operator or guidance, it is possible that reflected different variables to the settings or status of the device technology (e.g. quality). It is then possible to relate with each other.
- Procedures : The sequences of a process as provided corresponds only very rarely that transactions made by employees.
- Dependencies and stops time : The work activity may enroll in a timeframe more or less structured by the process, by advancing the work of other employees, or by events outside the company.
- The layout of the technical device : Often, initial plans of arrangement are now outdated. Indeed, subsequent implementations of equipment have been made.

Choice of the Situations to Analyze

It is rather difficult to extract a maxim or a rule in the choose of a situation that the ergonomist will do. The criteria he will use depending on the problem and the structure of the company. But it may be, for example, situations:

- Where complaints are most numerous
- Where the consequences are more serious

- Where the range of problems is the widest
- Playing a central role in the functioning of the company
- To be processing more or less long term

Analysis by the Activity

At first glance, each is tempted by the establishment of relations of direct causation between working conditions and health consequences or effectiveness. A noisy situation makes deaf, carrying heavy loads of produce musculoskeletal disorder, bad lighting, eyestrain, etc.. Unfortunately, this approach has important limitations: protection against noise may prohibit access to the machine, etc. ...

In fact, this approach neglects the fact that these relations necessarily pass through the activity of the employee. Indeed, it makes compromises with respect to constraints (it does not have them) to achieve the goals that are set and to limit the inconvenience caused by the tasks. For this reason, the ergonomist must focus its ergonomic analysis of work activity: it is in and by the activity of the operator in creating the effects of working conditions.

The role, in this context, analysis of the activity is not an evaluation (the workload for example) but the description and explanation of the mechanisms involved.

The Tools Available to the Ergonomist

The Observation

The observation is a specific feature in the Ergonomic analysis of work compared to other methods. This is to focus on the work as directed, whereas other approaches rely on "representations". Observation can be carried out openly or by focusing on the collection of certain categories of information with specific goals (we call then systematic observation).

- Broad observables categories : Travel, The direction of regards, Communications, Postures, The actions taken or information, Comments on the technical system and context, The collective
- Technical statement, there exist a variety of techniques to conduct surveys. The choice is made by the ergonomist in the constraints and circumstances. We'll list them here: The statements manuals, Video recordings, The Activity Chronic, The Metrics

The Verbalizations

To understand the activity, working conditions and their consequences, the verbalization of the employee is essential because: Activity can be reduced to what is observable;

The comments and actions take place at one moment, we must re-situate more broadly; The consequences of the activity are not all apparent.

However, there are limits to the verbalization to be taken into account:

- The employee described the work and its consequences in terms of what it believes to be the goals and interests of the speaker;
- The routine operations or learning old are not always mentioned spontaneously;
- Some aspects of the activities lend themselves well to verbal expression.

Participatory Ergonomics

Industrial Ergonomics programs seek to identify and correct factors that negatively impact the physical health of their workers. Participatory ergonomics programs seek to maximize the involvement of the workers in this process based on the simple fact that a worker is an expert on his or her job. The participatory approach to ergonomics relies on actively involving workers in implementing ergonomic knowledge, procedures and changes with the intention of improving working conditions, safety, productivity, quality, morale and/or comfort.

Implementing a Participatory Ergonomics Program in the Workplace

In order to determine if an ergonomics team/committee is right for a workplace, five factors need to be considered.

Resources and Support

A successful participatory ergonomics program requires initial and continuing resources and support from the top levels of management within the organization. The resources required include:

- time for the program to develop
- time to develop and implement solutions
- financial resources to make meaningful changes in the workplace
- management support for the individuals on the ergonomics team.

Ergo Team Formation

The ergonomics committee should be composed of people with the right mix of skills including technical or engineering knowledge, worker knowledge and input from an ergonomics expert. Successful, sustainable participatory ergonomics programs have an individual on the committee who takes on a leadership or "ergonomics champion" role .

Training Needs

Training principles and methods are central to the success of the participatory ergonomics process. Three major aspects of training should be considered early in the process of implementing a participatory ergonomics program. Initial training in ergonomics for committee members should include ergonomics concepts and tools. Training on topics such as meeting and project management may be beneficial, depending on the past experience of committee members with committee work and implementing change. Additionally, it is important for the workforce as a whole to gain an understanding of ergonomics to improve their support for the participatory ergonomics process.

Workplace Organization Factors

The research literature contains limited discussion of the effect of the organization's characteristics (culture) on the success of a participatory ergonomics intervention. The organizational climate and the timing of the introduction of the program can affect the outcome. Integrating the participatory ergonomics program into existing health and safety programs can increase the chances of success.

Involving the Workforce in Ergonomics

The ergonomics committee needs to respond to expectations about the ergonomics program. It is imperative to gain support or "buy in" from the workforce as most will not be directly involved with the ergonomics committee. The ergonomics program needs to be visible within the organization; this can be accomplished by ensuring that there is a focused effort to communicate with the workforce and by involving key stakeholders in all changes that are investigated and implemented.

Soft Ergonomics

Soft Ergonomics is the study of designing virtual interfaces that cater towards the wellness of the human body, its emotional and cognitive abilities.

Soft Ergonomics is a subset of Ergonomics and Human Factors Engineering, a larger body of the study of human abilities for designing equipment and devices that fit the human body. Soft Ergonomics can be thus defined as the ability of any virtual interface(computer application, website, ATM options, parking meter etc.) to make it comfortable for the user to use the interface while working on the user's request.

Overview

Soft Ergonomics only deals with virtual interfaces. It tries to find a compromise between user expectations, system workflow and aesthetics. Users from various cultural and technological background are exposed to a common interface. The interface developer seeks to ensure that the interface does not harm the user psychologically, physiologically or emotionally. Soft Ergonomics generally takes into account the following human factors when building a virtual interface:

1. Physical Limitations: Not all who use a virtual interface are physically equal. If the designed interface only caters to right-handed individuals, or people within a certain height range then the interface might need a redesign. One of the leading discussion is with respect to visually impaired users.

2. Cognitive Abilities: If the product(software application, website) is designed for any casual user, then the designer should not expect that all users would be experts, with high cognitive abilities. The usage of the application should not need the user to know a lot of information prior to using the interface. For example, using an automated teller machine can require memorizing a pin number but not the account number.

3. Emotional Needs: The interface should be 'designed for the occasion' or context. It should not leave the user confused, either how to start using the interface or what to do when an error occurs. Confusion leads to frustration, which eventually builds stress in the body causing long term emotional damage.

Criteria for Soft Ergonomics

The following lists(non-exhaustive) some of the most common criteria for evaluating soft ergonomics.

1. Consistency: The design should be consistent across the entire application. Consistent sequence of actions, identical terminologies and platform conventions should be followed throughout the application.

2. Efficiency: The virtual interface should allow efficient use of user's time. The screens should load and display content within acceptable amount of time. The more than expected time a user has to wait, more stress is built into the human body causing long term damage. The interface should also have functionality for advanced users. While being non-obtrusive to novice users, accelerators or shortcuts should be available for experienced users.

3. Design: The system should preferably have minimalistic and aesthetically pleasing design. While this has no direct relation to the product or task in hand, minimalistic design help user easily consume the data and hence there is less stress on the human

mind and aesthetically pleasing design increases the 'feel good' factor in the user. Following the principles of contrast, repetition, alignment and proximity will also help as they come naturally to humans.

4. Memory: User's memory load should be minimized. All information that a user needs from the application to perform a task should be presented or easily retrievable by the user.

5. Context Help: While the 'Help' menu and options should be non obstructive to the user, context help should be always available to the user.

References

- "Tallest Man". Guinness World Records. March 19, 2010. Archived from the original on March 19, 2010. Retrieved 2010-03-19. at Wayback machine
- Haines, H.; Wilson, J. R.; Vink, P.; Koningsveld, E. (2002). "Validating a framework for participatory ergonomics (the PEF)". Ergonomics. 45 (4): 309–327. PMID 12028727. doi:10.1080/00140130210123516
- Jain, Anil K.; Ross, Arun (2008). "Introduction to Biometrics". In Jain, AK; Flynn; Ross, A. Handbook of Biometrics. Springer. pp. 1–22. ISBN 978-0-387-71040-2
- "Lighting Ergonomics - General" by Canadian Centre for Occupational Health & Safety, CCOHS, January, 2003, retrieved November 3, 2007
- Chen, J.; Gefen, A.; Greenstein, A.; Matzkin, H.; Elad, D. (2000). "Predicting penile size during erection". International Journal of Impotence Research. 12 (6): 328–333. PMID 11416836. doi:10.1038/sj.ijir.3900627
- Allen, JS; Damasio H; Grabowski TJ (2002). "Normal neuroanatomical variation in the human brain: An MRI-volumetric study". Am J Phys Anthropol. 118 (4): 341–58. PMID 12124914. doi:10.1002/ajpa.10092
- Chivers, Tom (2009-09-24). "Human extremes: the tallest, shortest, heaviest and lightest people ever". The Telegraph. Retrieved 2013-05-26
- Nagamachi, M. (1995). "Requisites and practices of participatory ergonomics". International Journal of Industrial Ergonomics. 15 (5): 371–377. doi:10.1016/0169-8141(94)00082-E
- Illuminating Engineering Society of North America. RIESNA Lighting Handbook. (9th ed.). Illuminating Engineering Society of North America. ISBN 0-87995-150-8
- International Ergonomics Association. What is Ergonomics Archived May 20, 2013, at the Wayback Machine.. Website. Retrieved 6 December 2010
- Jain A.; Hong L.; Pankanti S. (2000). "Biometric Identification" (PDF). Communications of the ACM. 43 (2): 91–98. doi:10.1145/328236.328110
- Kuorinka, I.; Patry, L. (1995). "Participation as a means of promoting occupational health. International Journal of Industrial". Ergonomics. 15 (5): 365–370. doi:10.1016/0169-8141(94)00083-F
- "Biometrics: Overview". Biometrics.cse.msu.edu. 6 September 2007. Archived from the original on 2012-01-07. Retrieved 2012-06-10

2

Understanding Cognitive Ergonomics

Cognitive ergonomics studies mental processes like memory, perception and motor response. It studies human strategies devised as a response to a work process. The significant themes related to the subject matter are decision-making, work stress, workload, skilled performance and human reliability. The chapter serves as a source to understand cognitive ergonomics.

Cognitive Ergonomics

Cognitive ergonomics, defined by the International Ergonomics Association "is concerned with mental processes, such as perception, memory, reasoning, and motor response, as they affect interactions among humans and other elements of a system. The relevant topics include mental workload, decision-making, skilled performance, human-computer interaction, human reliability, work stress and training as these may relate to human-system design." Cognitive ergonomics studies cognition in work and operational settings, in order to optimize human well-being and system performance. It is a subset of the larger field of human factors and ergonomics.

Goals

Cognitive ergonomics (sometimes known as cognitive engineering though this was an earlier field) is an emerging branch of ergonomics which places particular emphasis on the analysis of cognitive processes required of operators in modern industries and similar milieus. Examples include diagnosis, workload, situation awareness, decision making, and planning. Cognitive ergonomics aims at enhancing performance of cognitive tasks by means of several interventions, including these:

- user-centered design of human-machine interaction and human-computer interaction (HCI);
- design of information technology systems that support cognitive tasks (e.g., cognitive artifacts);
- development of training programs;
- work redesign to manage cognitive workload and increase human reliability.

History

The field of cognitive ergonomics emerged predominantly in the 70's with the advent of the personal computer and new developments in the fields of cognitive psychology and artificial intelligence. CE contrasts the tradition of physical ergonomics because "cognitive ergonomics is...the application of psychology to work...to achieve the optimization between people and their work." Viewed as an applied science, the methods involved with creating cognitive ergonomic design have changed with the rapid development in technological advances over the last 27 years. In the 80's, there was a worldwide transition in the methodological approach to design. According to van der Veer, Enid Mumford was one of the pioneers of interactive systems engineering, and advocated the notion of user-centered design, wherein the user is considered and "included in all phases of the design".

There are several different models which describe the criteria for designing user-friendly technology. A number of models focus on a systematic process for design, using task analysis to evaluate the cognitive processes involved with a given task and develop adequate interface capabilities. Task analysis in past research has focused on the evaluation of cognitive task demands, concerning motor control and cognition during visual tasks such as operating machinery, or the evaluation of attention and focus via the analysis of eye saccades of pilots when flying. Neuroergonomics, a subfield of cognitive ergonomics, aims to enhance human-computer interaction by using neural correlates to better understand situational task demands. Neuroergonomic research at the university of Iowa has been involved with assessing safe-driving protocol, enhancing elderly mobility, and analyzing cognitive abilities involved with the navigation of abstract virtual environments."

Methods

Successful, ergonomic intervention in the area of cognitive tasks requires a thorough understanding not only of the demands of the work situation, but also of user strategies in performing cognitive tasks and of limitations in human cognition. In some cases, the artifacts or tools used to carry out a task may impose their own constraints and limitations (e.g., navigating through a large number of GUI screens). Tools may also co-determine the very nature of the task. In this sense, the analysis of cognitive tasks should examine both the interaction of users with their work setting and the user interaction with artifacts or tools; the latter is very important as modern artifacts (e.g., control panels, software, expert systems) become increasingly sophisticated. Emphasis lies on how to design human-machine interfaces and cognitive artifacts so that human performance is sustained in work environments where information may be unreliable, events may be difficult to predict, multiple simultaneous goals may be in conflict, and performance may be time constrained.

User Interface Modeling

Cognitive Task Analysis

Cognitive task analysis is a general term for the set of methods used to identify the mental demands and cognitive skills needed to complete a task. Frameworks like GOMS provide a formal set of methods for identifying the mental activities required by a task and an artifact, such as a desktop computer system. By identifying the sequence of mental activities of a user engaged in a task, cognitive ergonomics engineers can identify bottlenecks and critical paths that may present opportunities for improvement or risks (such as human error) that merit changes in training or system behavior.

Computer-Aided Ergonomics

Computer-aided ergonomics is an engineering discipline using computers to solve complex ergonomic problems involving interaction between the human body and its environment. The human body holds a great complexity thus it can be beneficial to use computers to solve problems involving the human body and the environment that surrounds it.

Overview

Computer-aided ergonomics is an interdisciplinary field of work that involves the use of a computer to solve complex problems regarding a human body interacting with an environment. As the title reveals, having a computer to help find the best ergonomic solution in a given situation. Ergonomics traditionally involves many disciplines including biomechanics, anthropometry, mechanical engineering, industrial engineering, kinesiology, health sciences and physiology. Due to the highly interdisciplinary and complex nature of ergonomics it is hard to get a full understanding of a situation. As the human body is a complex system, thus it is beneficial to have a computer system that models the human body as a mechanical system. The human body contains several parts that can be modeled as known mechanical systems, for example bones connected with joints and driven by actuators (muscles).

Example of a System

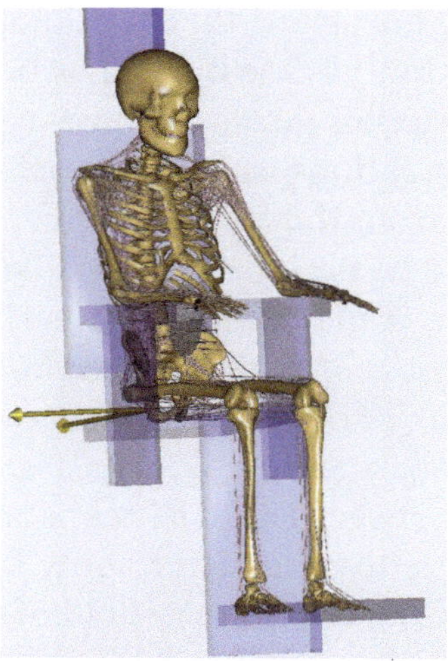

Example of a skeletal mannequin

One example of a computer system that can be used as a computer-aided ergonomics system is that consider the human body as a dynamic multi-rigid-body system. The human model is a public domain model contains most of the bones, muscles and joints that are present in the human body. The model in total have more than 1000 muscle elements, and many muscle elements have been modeled with the most detailed muscle model theory described by Hill, A.V. in 1938. The muscle model contains information as physiological cross-sectional area, length, penation angle, ratio of red and white fibers and so on. The AnyBody modeling system is capable of modeling almost any human voluntary movement or static situation. One example of a model, could be a seated model, where the human body is placed in a chair, that have a seat, backrest, headrest, leg rest, footrest, and armrest. The model can then calculate the forces acting between the human body and the chair, as well as for example the forces between any given spinal vertebra. This could be used for finding the optimal seated posture for a person, who suffers from lower back pain, assuming that greater load on a vertebra result in greater pain.

Benefits of Computer-aided Ergonomics

The question is "In what scenario" it would be beneficial to use computer-aided ergonomics compared to traditional ergonomics. First of all computer aided ergonomics using for example a musculo-skeletal modeling system as The [AnyBody Modeling system], would be beneficial in physical ergonomics, which traditional combines aspects from the human anatomical, anthropometric, physiological and biomechanical characteristics related to some physical activity. The model can provide a quantitative foundation for ergonomic design and recommendations. Traditionally "Ergonomics" has been based on recommendations derived from empirical data from various working tasks; if many people get injured from working in a certain posture, it is recommended to avoid working in that posture. However, when applying the recommendations to another related working posture, the posture or the movement often does not match exactly. This means that the theory and recommendations does not apply to the new situation. In this case it could be beneficial to model the situation in order to find out how the reaction forces and muscle activities differ from the first situation, where the recommendations were based on empirical data. A combination of risk factors can be derived from the model output. For example, when designing an office chair, one would like to design it to fulfill several demands; comfortable, relaxing, supporting and so on. Some of the criteria related to the demands might be conflicting for example; comfort is often related to the shear force on the seat, which should be kept as low as possible. The seat shear force could be removed by making a horizontal seat and rising the backrest to 90 degrees however this would not be relaxing. Therefore, a combination of seat and backrest angles needs to be considered in order to find optimal seated postures related to only the two design variables. Computer-aided ergonomics is an interdisciplinary field of work, that involve the use of a computer to solve complex problems that involve a person interacting with an environment. As the title reveals, it is all about having a computer to help finding the best ergonomic solution. Ergonomics involves many disciplines, such as biomechanics, anthropometry, mechanical engineering, industrial engineering, kinesiology, health sciences and physiology. Due to the highly interdisciplinary it is hard to get a full understanding of a situation based on knowledge, unless the knowledge in some way is built into a computer system.

User Interface Modeling

User interface modeling is a development technique used by computer application programmers. Today's user interfaces (UIs) are complex software components, which play an essential role in the usability of an application. The development of UIs requires therefore, not only guidelines and best practice reports, but also a development process including the elaboration of visual models and a standardized notation for this visualization.

The term *user interface modeling* is mostly used in an information technology context. A user interface model is a representation of how the end user(s) interact with a computer program or another device and also how the system responds. The modeling task is then to show all the "*directly experienced* aspects of a thing or device" [Trætteberg2002].

Modeling user interfaces is a well-established discipline in its own right. For example, modeling techniques can describe interaction objects, tasks, and lower-level dialogs in user interfaces. Using models as part of user interface development can help capture user requirements, avoid premature commitment to specific layouts and widgets, and make the relationships between an interface's different parts and their roles explicit. [SilvaPaton2003].

Languages

MARIA

MARIA XML (Model-based lAnguage foR Interactive Applications) is a universal, declarative, multiple abstraction level, XML-based user interface markup language for modelling interactive applications in ubiquitous environments.

UML

Some aspects of user interface modeling can be realized using UML. However, the language is not mainly intended for this kind of modeling, which may render the models somewhat synthetic.

UMLi

UMLi is an extension of UML, and adds support for representation commonly occurring in user interfaces.

Because application models in UML describe few aspects of user interfaces, and because the model-based user interface development environments (MB-UIDE) lack ability for modeling applications, the University of Manchester started the research project UMLi in 1998. UMLi aims to address this problem of designing and implementing user interfaces using a combination of UML and MB-UIDE.

UsiXML

UsiXML (USer Interface eXtensible Markup Language) is an XML-based specification language for user interface design. It supports the description of UI for multiple contexts of use such as Character User Interfaces (CUIs), Graphical User Interfaces (GUIs), Auditory User Interfaces, and Multimodal User Interfaces.

DiaMODL

DiaMODL combines a dataflow-oriented language (Pisa interactor abstraction) with UML Statecharts which has focus on behavior. It is capable of modeling the dataflow as well as the behavior of interaction objects. It may be used for documenting the function and structure of concrete user interfaces.

Himalia

Himalia combines the Hypermedia Models with the control/composite paradigm. It is a full user interface language, it may be used for specifying but also for running it, because of this the designer tool can categorized as a guilder.

Model Types

The different aspects of a user interface requires different model types. Some of the models that may be considered for UI-modeling are:

- Domain model, including data model (defines the objects that a user can view, access and manipulate through the user interface)
- Navigation model, defines how the objects that a user view could be navigated through the user interface
- Task model. (describes the tasks an end user performs and dictates what interaction capabilities must be designed)
- User model (represents the different characteristics of end users and the roles they are playing within the organization)
- Platform model (used to model the physical devices that are intended to host the application and how they interact with each other)

- Dialogue model (how users can interact with the objects presentation (as push buttons, commands, etc.), with interaction media (as voice input, touch screen, etc.) and the reactions that the user interface communicates via these objects)
- Presentation model (application appearance, representation of the visual, haptic and auditory elements that the user interface offers to its users)
- Application model (commands and data the application provides)

UML can be used for several of the models mentioned above with varying degree of success, but it lacks support for user modeling, platform modeling and presentation model.

Approaches

There exist several approaches to modeling a user interface.

Usage-centered Design

In usage-centered design, the modeling task is to show how the actual presentation of a planned system and how the user interaction is supposed to happen. This is probably the most praised approach, and it has been used successfully on a variety of small and large-scale projects. Its strengths are in complex problems.

Alternative Approaches to Model-based UIs

The know issue of model-based approaches is information restatement and lack of mechanisms effectively to solve cross-cutting concerns [Cerny2013]. Model-based solution work well on their own, but integration with alternative approaches bring complexity in development and maintenance efforts.

Code-inspection Based

These approaches bases on existing general purpose language (GPL) code base [Cerny2012]. They inspect the code through meta-programming and assemble a structural model that is transformed to the UI. This approach addresses information restatement. These approaches does not fit to adaptive and context-aware UIs.

Generative Programming

These approaches connect domain methods with GPL [Generative programming]. They address cross-cutting concerns although only at compile-time, which does not fit to future adaptive UIs that need runtime information.

Aspect-based UIs

Aspect-based solution suggested by [Cerny2013][Cerny2013a][AspectFaces] integrates advantages of code-inspection based and generative programming approaches. It inspects existing code and applies aspect oriented methods to address cross-cutting concerns. It works at runtime, reduces information restatement and at the same time separates UI concerns which allows to reuse each independent of others. In the study at [Cerny2013] authors reduce UI code by 32% through aspect=based UI approach applied to a production system. Main advantages are templating for adjusting the presentation, separate definitions of concerns and mostly generic transformation rules applicable across various data.

Content Models

Models of this kind show the contents of a user interface and its different components. Aesthetics and behavior details are not included in this kind of models as it is in usage-centered design models.

Task Analysis

Task analysis is the analysis of how a task is accomplished, including a detailed description of both manual and mental activities, task and element durations, task frequency, task allocation, task complexity, environmental conditions, necessary clothing and equipment, and any other unique factors involved in or required for one or more people to perform a given task.

Information from a task analysis can then be used for many purposes, such as personnel selection and training, tool or equipment design, procedure design (e.g., design of checklists or decision support systems) and automation. Though distinct, task analysis is related to user analysis.

Applications

The term “task” is often used interchangeably with activity or process. Task analysis often results in a hierarchical representation of what steps it takes to perform a task for which there is a goal and for which there is some lowest-level “action” or interaction among humans and/or machines: this is known as hierarchical task analysis. Tasks may be identified and defined at multiple levels of abstraction as required to support the purpose of the analysis. A critical task analysis, for example, is an analysis of human performance requirements which, if not accomplished in accordance with system requirements, will likely have adverse effects on cost, system reliability, efficiency, effectiveness, or safety. Task analysis is often performed by human factors and ergonomics professionals.

Task analysis may be of manual tasks, such as bricklaying, and be analyzed as time and motion studies using concepts from industrial engineering. Cognitive task analysis is applied to modern work environments such as supervisory control where little physical work occurs, but the tasks are more related to situation assessment, decision making, and response planning and execution.

Task analysis is also used in education. It is a model that is applied to classroom tasks to discover which curriculum components are well matched to the capabilities of students with learning disabilities and which task modification might be necessary. It discovers which tasks a person hasn't mastered, and the information processing demands of tasks that are easy or problematic. In behavior modification, it is a breakdown of a complex behavioral sequence into steps. This often serves as the basis for chaining.

The results of task analysis are often represented in task models, which clearly indicate the relations among the various tasks, An example notation used to specify task models is ConcurTaskTrees (by Fabio Paternò), which is also supported by tools that are freely available.

Versus work Domain Analysis

If task analysis is likened to a set of instructions on how to navigate from Point A to Point B, then Work domain analysis (WDA) is like having a map of the terrain that includes Point A and Point B. WDA is broader and focuses on the environmental constraints and opportunities for behavior, as in Gibsonian ecological psychology and ecological interface design (Vicente, 1999; Bennett & Flach, 2011, p. 61)

Documentation

Since the 1980s, a major change in technical documentation has been to emphasize the tasks performed with a system rather than documenting the system itself. In software documentation particularly, long printed technical manuals that exhaustively describe every function of the software are being replaced by online help organized into tasks. This is part of the new emphasis on usability and user-centered design rather than system/software/product design.

This task orientation in technical documentation began with publishing guidelines issued by IBM in the late 1980s. Later IBM studies led to John Carroll's theory of minimalism in the 1990s.

With the development of XML as a markup language suitable for both print and online documentation (replacing SGML with its focus on print), IBM developed the Darwin Information Typing Architecture XML standard in 2000. Now an OASIS standard, DITA has a strong emphasis on task analysis. Its three basic information types are Task, Concept, and Reference. Tasks are analyzed into steps, with a main goal of identifying steps that are reusable in multiple tasks.

Hierarchical Task Analysis

Hierarchical task analysis (HTA) is a task description method and a variant of task analysis. Task description is a necessary precursor for other analysis techniques, including critical path analysis (CPA). HTA is used to produce an exhaustive description of tasks in a hierarchical structure of goals, sub-goals, operations and plans. In HTA, tasks are broken down into progressively smaller units.

Operations and Plans

Operations are the actions performed by people interacting with a system or by the system itself, and plans explain the conditions necessary for these operations. Operations describe the smallest individual task steps in the HTA, i.e. those which cannot be broken down into plans and further operations. They are the individual actions, such as 'visually locate control' or 'move hand to control', which the user must perform in a particular combination to achieve the goal of task completion.

Applying

The following steps should be followed when conducting a HTA:

1. Define the task under investigation and identify the purpose of the task analysis. The analyst should have some further evaluation methods in mind for which the HTA will be useful and should have reason for needing this type of analysis to be performed.
2. Data collection – In order to carry out the HTA it is necessary to obtain data on how the task is performed. This could be collected via observation of the task in question or from a detailed specification of the device under analysis. Alternatively, interviews or questionnaires with people that have first-hand experience of performing that task could be conducted to gather the necessary detail.
3. Define the overall task goal, which will be presented as the top level in the HTA. An example might be "increase fan speed by two steps". This describes what is being achieved by performing the task; however, at this stage there is no indication of how the task will be performed.
4. Determine the next level of sub-goals by breaking down the overall goal. A sub-goal for the above example might be "open the climate menu". This provides more information about how to accomplish the task; however, it can still be broken down into smaller units, which will describe the individual operations (performed via the visual, manual or cognitive modes) that need to be performed.
5. Continue breaking down the sub-goals until all operations are identified. Operations in the "reduce fan speed task" will include "move finger to climate menu button" and "touch climate menu button".

6. Define plans to describe how to perform the operations in each sub-goal level of the hierarchy. In the fan speed example, the two operations will have to be performed in series, one after the other. The plan will instruct the user to "perform 1, then 2". Operations can also be performed in parallel, and in this case the plan would instruct the user to "perform 1 and 2 together". Numbers should be assigned to the different levels in the hierarchy.

Organising the Hierarchy

Each level in the HTA should be numbered according to its hierarchical level: The overall goal is the highest hierarchical level and should be numbered 0. The first sub-goal in the hierarchy will be 1, also with plan 1. Further levels just extend this system - third hierarchical level: 1.1, fourth hierarchical level: 1.1.1, and so on. A HTA can be represented in list or diagram form. In list form lines should be indented to denote the different hierarchical levels. In diagram form each operation should be placed within a box and links should be made between them: a lower hierarchical level should branch from underneath a higher level operation. Plans should be written next to the branches to describe the way in which the branched operations should be carried out.

Applications and Limitations

HTA is a task description method which is most commonly used as a starting point for further analyses such as multimodal CPA and SHERPA. On its own, HTA does not provide results for usability evaluation; however, you should be able to study the HTA in order to learn about the structure of different tasks. It may also allow you to highlight unnecessary task steps or potential errors that might occur in task performance. HTA is a fairly time-consuming method to carry out as each individual operation in a task needs to be analysed; however, creating a comprehensive HTA can considerably reduce the time required for other modelling methods.

Neuroergonomics

Neuroergonomics is the application of neuroscience to ergonomics. Traditional ergonomic studies rely predominantly on psychological explanations to address human factors issues such as: work performance, operational safety, and workplace-related risks (e.g., repetitive stress injuries). Neuroergonomics, in contrast, addresses the biological substrates of ergonomic concerns, with an emphasis on the role of the human nervous system.

Overview

Neuroergonomics has two major aims: to use existing/emerging knowledge of human performance and brain function to design systems for safer and more efficient operation, and to advance this understanding of the relationship between brain function and performance in real-world tasks.

To meet these goals, neuroergonomics combines two disciplines—neuroscience, the study of brain function, and human factors, the study of how to match technology with the capabilities and limitations of people so they can work effectively and safely. The goal of merging these two fields is to use the startling discoveries of human brain and physiological functioning both to inform the design of technologies in the workplace and home, and to provide new training methods that enhance performance, expand capabilities, and optimize the fit between people and technology.

Research in the area of neuroergonomics has blossomed in recent years with the emergence of noninvasive techniques for monitoring human brain function that can be used to study various aspects of human behavior in relation to technology and work, including mental workload, visual attention, working memory, motor control, human-automation interaction, and adaptive automation. Consequently, this interdisciplinary field is concerned with investigations of the neural bases of human perception, cognition, and performance in relation to systems and technologies in the real world—for example, in the use of computers and various other machines at home or in the workplace, and in operating vehicles such as aircraft, cars, trains, and ships.

Some studies have shown the promise of using transcranial magnetic stimulation (TMS) and transcranial direct-current stimulation (tDCS) to improve cognitive skills during tasks. While initially used to treat various neurological disorders such as Parkinson's disease or dementia, the scope of TMS is expanding. In TMS, electricity is passed through a magnetic coil that is positioned near the person's scalp. Results from studies show that noninvasive brain stimulation leads to 20 more minutes of sustained vigilance performance.

Neuroimaging & Mental Workload

A major component of neuroergonomic studies has been neuroimaging. There are two ways that neuroimaging methods are used. The first way is to display cerebral metabolic processes associated with neural activity with the use of a functional MRI (fMRI) and transcranial Doppler (TCD) sonography. An fMRI allows for researchers to localize neural activity within the brain. One of the major advantages of fMRI is the fact that it is a noninvasive imaging method. Before the invention of the fMRI, methods such as positron emission tomography required the injection of a radioactive tracer. The second way that neuroimaging is used is to identify the timing of neural processing, with the use of electroencephalography (EEG) and event-related potentials (ERPs).

Using an fMRI, mental workload can be quantified by an increase in cerebral blood flow in regions of the prefrontal cortex (PFC). Many fMRI studies show that there is increased PFC activation during a working memory task. Equally important as measuring mental workload, is evaluating the operator vigilance, or attentiveness. Using TCD to monitor blood flow velocity in intercranial arteries, it was shown that a decrease in blood flow was associated with a decrease in vigilance and depletion of cognitive resources.

Adaptive Automation

Adaptive automation, a novel neuroergonomic concept, refers to a human-machine system that uses real-time assessment of the operator's workload to make the necessary changes to enhance performance. For adaptive automation to work, the system must utilize an accurate operator-state classifier for the real-time assessment. Operator-state classifiers such as discriminant analysis and artificial neural networks show an accuracy of 70% to 85% in real-time. An important part to properly implementing adaptive automation is figuring out how big a workload needs to be to require intervention. Implementing neuroergonomic adaptive automation would require the development of nonintrusive sensors and even techniques to track eye movement. Current research into assessing a person's mental state includes using facial electromyography to detect confusion.

Experiments show that a human-robot team performs better at controlling air and ground vehicles than either a human or robot (i.e. the automatic target recognition system). When compared to 100% human control and static automation, participants showed higher trust and self-confidence, as well as lower perceived workload, when using adaptive automation.

In adaptive automation, getting the machine to accurately reason how to respond to the changes and get back to peak performance is the biggest challenge. The machine has to be able to determine to what extent it must make the changes. This is also a consequence of the complexity of the system and factors such as: how easily can the sensed parameter be quantified, how many parameters in the machine's system can be changed, and how well can these different machine parameters be coordinated.

Brain Computer Interfaces

A developing area of research called brain-computer interfaces (BCIs) strives to use different types of brain signals to operate external devices, without any motor input from the person. BCIs provide promise for patients with limited motor capabilities, such as those with amyotrophic lateral sclerosis. When the user engages in a specific mental activity, it generates a unique brain electrical potential that is processed and relayed into a signal for the external device. BCIs using signals from EEGs and ERPs have been used to operate voice synthesizers and move robotic arms. Research for BCIs began in the 1970s at the University of California Los Angeles, and its current focus is towards neuroprosthetic applications. BCIs can be substantially improved by incorporating high-level control, context, the environment, as well as virtual reality into its design.

Applications in Stroke Rehabilitation

As of 2011, there has been an effort to applying a rehabilitation robot connected to a non-invasive brain-computer interface to promote brain plasticity and motor learning following a stroke. Half of stroke survivors experience unilateral paralysis or weakness, and approximately 30-60% of them do not regain function. Typical treatment, post-stroke, involves constraint-induced movement therapy and robotic therapy, which work to restore motor activity by forcing the movement of the weak limbs. Current active therapy cannot be utilized by patients who suffer complete control loss or paralysis, and do not have any residual motor ability to work with.

With a focus on these underserved patients, a BCI was created that used the electrical brain signals detected by an EEG to control an upper-limb rehabilitative robot. The user is instructed to imagine the motor activity while the EEG picks up the associated brain signals. The BCI uses a linear transformation algorithm to convert the EEG spectral features into commands for the robot. An experiment done on 24 subjects tested a non-BCI group, which used sensorimotor rhythms to control the robot, against the BCI-group, which used the BCI-robot system. The results from the brain-plasticity analysis showed that there was a decrease in beta wave activity in the subjects of the BCI-group, which is associated with a change in movement. The results also showed that the BCI-group performed better than the non-BCI group in every measure for motor learning.

Virtual Reality

Virtual reality could allow for testing how human operators would work in dangerous environments without actually putting them in harm's way. For example, it would allow the testing of how fatigue or a new technology would affect a driver or a pilot in their specific environment, without the possibility of injury. Being able to evaluate the effects of some new workplace technology in virtual reality, before real life implementation, could save money and lives. Bringing virtual reality technology to the point where it can accurately mimic real life is difficult, but its potential is vast.

Healthcare Training

Healthcare training programs have adopted virtual reality simulation (VRS) as a training tool for nursing students. This computer-based three-dimensional simulation tool allows for nursing students to practice various nursing skills repeatedly in a risk-free environment. A nursing program at a major Midwestern state university agreed to utilize a VRS module for teaching the insertion of an intravenous (IV) catheter, and complete an evaluation on the effectiveness of the program. The VRS composed of a computer program and a haptic arm device, which worked together to simulate the feel of vascular access. On the computer screen, the user would have to select the equipment for the procedure in the correct order. The user then palpates the veins of the haptic arm, and virtually inserts the IV catheter. The program provides immediate feedback by notifying the user when he/she misses a step and needs to restart the procedure.

Results of evaluation pointed to the VRS an "excellent learning tool" for increasing a student's knowledge on the procedure. All eight of the nursing faculty who participated agreed to this much, and that they would recommend that students work with the VRS before performing the IV catheter insertion on real patients.

This tool allows educators to expose students to an extensive range of real-life patient conditions and nursing experiences. The central advantage of the VRS program is the availability of a variety of case scenarios, which allow students to increase their awareness of differences in patient responses to IV catheter insertion. From the standpoint of the student, the virtual reality simulation helps bridge the gap between nursing theory and practice.

Applications for Neurocognitive Disabilities

Neuroergonomic assessments have tremendous potential for evaluating the psychomotor performance in an individual with a neurocognitive disability or following a stroke or surgery. They would allow for a standardized method for measuring the change in neurocognitive function during rehabilitation for a neurocognitive disability. In terms of rehabilitation, it would allow for the efforts to be goal-oriented. These tests could be applied for measuring change following operational procedures such as neurosurgery, carotid endarterectomy, and coronary artery bypass graft.

Applications for Driving Safety

One of the main application domains of neuroergonomics is driving safety, especially for older drivers with cognitive impairments. Driving requires the integration of multiple cognitive processes, which can be studied separately if the right kinds of tools are used. The types of tools used to evaluate cognition during driving include driving simulators, instrumented vehicles, and part task simulators.

The Crossmodal Research Laboratory in Oxford is working on developing a system of warning signals to grab the attention of a distracted driver, in an effort to make driving safer for everybody. The research has found that using auditory icons, such as a car horn, is a better warning signal than a pure tone. On top of that, spatial auditory cues work better at redirecting the driver's attention than non-spatialized auditory cues. Cues that integrate multiple senses, such as an audiotactile signal, grab attention better than unisensory cues.

References

- Van der veer GC (2008). "Cognitive Ergonomics in Interface Design – Discussion of a Moving Science". journal of universal computer science. 14 (16): 2614–2629

- [Cerny2012] – T. Cerny and E. Song. Model-driven Rich Form Generation. Information: An International Interdisciplinary Journal, 15(7, SI):2695--2714, JUL 2012
- Lee JD (2001). "Emerging challenges in cognitive ergonomics: managing swarms of self-organizing agent-based automation". Theoretical Issues in ergonomic science. 2 (3): 238–250. doi:10.1080/14639220110104925
- De Visser, E., & Parasuraman, R. (2011). Adaptive aiding of human-robot teaming: Effects of imperfect automation on performance, trust, and workload. Journal Of Cognitive Engineering And Decision Making, 5(2), 209-231
- Hutton RJB, Militello LG (1998). "applied cognitive task analysis (ACTA): a practitioner's toolkit for understanding cognitive task demands". Ergonomics. 41 (11): 1618–1641. doi:10.1080/001401398186108
- Allison, B., Leeb, R., Brunner, C., Muller-Putz, G., Bauernfeind, G., Kelly, J., & Neuper, C. (n.d). Toward smarter BCIs: extending BCIs through hybridization and intelligent control. Journal Of Neural Engineering, 9(1)
- Wilson, K. M., Helton, W. S., & Wiggins, M. W. (2013). Cognitive engineering. Wiley Interdisciplinary Reviews: Cognitive Science, 4(1), 17-31.doi:10.1002/wcs.1204
- Henry J., M., & David J., M. (n.d). Neurocognitive disability, stroke, and surgery: A role for neuroergonomics?. Journal Of Psychosomatic Research, 63, 613-615
- "Cognitive ergonomics - past, present, future: 10 lessons learned (10 lessons remaining) Proceedings of the Human Factors and Ergonomics Society ... Annual Meeting". human factors and ergonomics society. June 6, 2010. Retrieved November 26, 2011
- Lees, M. N., Cosman, J. D., Lee, J. D., Fricke, N., & Rizzo, M. (2010). Translating cognitive neuroscience to the driver's operational environment: A neuroergonomic approach. American Journal Of Psychology, 123(4), 391-411

3

Occupational Hazards and Safety

Occupational hazards are threats faced by workers in their workplace. It includes hazards such as biological hazards, psychosocial hazards, chemical hazards and physical hazards. The chapter strategically encompasses and incorporates the major components and key concepts of occupational hazards and safety, providing a complete understanding.

Occupational Hazard

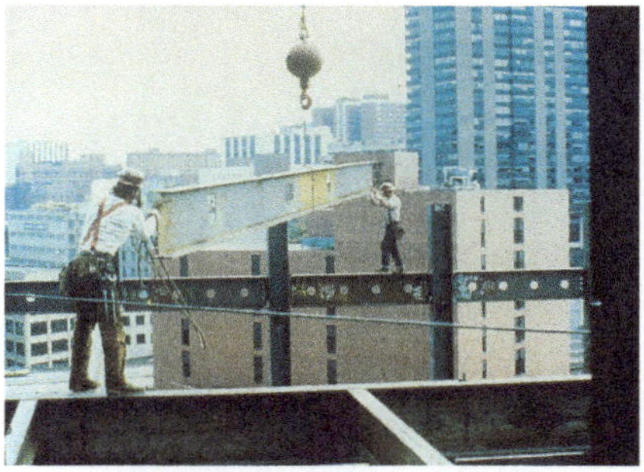

At-risk workers without appropriate safety equipment

An occupational hazard is a hazard experienced in the workplace. Occupational hazards can encompass many types of hazards, including chemical hazards, biological hazards (biohazards), psychosocial hazards, and physical hazards. In the United States, the National Institute for Occupational Safety and Health (NIOSH) conduct workplace investigations and research addressing workplace health and safety hazards resulting in guidelines. The Occupational Safety and Health Administration (OSHA) establishes enforceable standards to prevent workplace injuries and illnesses. In the EU a similar role is taken by EU-OSHA.

Occupational hazard as a term signifies both long-term and short-term risks associated with the workplace environment and is a field of study within occupational safety and health and public health. Short term risks may include physical injury, while long-term risks may be increased risk of developing cancer or heart disease.

Chemical Hazards

Chemical hazards are a subtype of occupational hazards that involve dangerous chemicals. Exposure to chemicals in the workplace can cause acute or long-term detrimental health effects. There are many classifications of hazardous chemicals, including neurotoxins, immune agents, dermatologic agents, carcinogens, reproductive toxins, systemic toxins, asthmagens, pneumoconiotic agents, and sensitizers.

NIOSH sets recommended exposure limits (REL's) as well as recommends preventative measures on specific chemicals in order to reduce or eliminate negative health effects from exposure to those chemicals. Additionally, NIOSH keeps an index of chemical hazards based on their chemical name, Chemical Abstracts Service Registry Number (CAS No.), and RTECS Number.

This is evidence that workplace exposure to hazards such as silica dust, engine exhausts or welding fumes, among others are associated with increased prevalence of heart disease. Other workplace hazards have been shown to increase risk of pulmonary heart disease, stroke, and high blood pressure.

Biological Hazards

Biological agents, including microorganisms and toxins produced by living organisms, can cause health problems in workers. Influenza is an example of a biohazard which affects a broad population of workers.

Those who work outdoors encounter numerous biological hazards, including bites and stings from insects, spiders, snakes and scorpions, contact dermatitis from exposure to urushiol from poisonous *Toxicodendron* plants, Lyme disease, West Nile virus, and coccidioidomycosis. According to NIOSH, outdoor workers at risk for these hazards "include farmers, foresters, landscapers, groundskeepers, gardeners, painters, roofers, pavers, construction workers, laborers, mechanics, and any other workers who spend time outside."

Health care professionals are at risk to exposure to blood-borne illnesses (such as HIV, hepatitis B, and hepatitis C) and particularly to emerging infectious diseases, especially when not enough resources are available to control the spread of the disease. Veterinary health workers, including veterinarians, are at risk for exposure to zoonotic disease. Those who do clinical work in the field or in a laboratory risk exposure to West Nile virus if performing necropsies on birds affected by the virus or are otherwise working with infected tissue.

Other occupations at risk to biological hazard exposure include poultry workers, who are exposed to bacteria; and tattooists and piercers, who risk exposure to blood-borne pathogens.

Psychosocial Hazards

Psychosocial hazards are occupational hazards that affect someone's social life or psychological health. Psychosocial hazards in the workplace include occupational burnout and occupational stress, which can lead to burnout.

Physical Hazards

Physical hazards are a subtype of occupational hazards that involve environmental hazards that can cause harm with or without contact. Physical hazards include ergonomic hazards, radiation, heat and cold stress, vibration hazards, and noise hazards.

Noise

Each year in the US, twenty-two million workers are exposed to noise levels that could potentially harm their health. Occupational hearing loss is the most common occupational illness in the manufacturing sector. Workers in certain fields, such as musicians, mine workers, and even those involved with stock car racing, are exposed to higher levels of noise and therefore are at a higher risk of developing hearing loss.

While permanent, noise-induced hearing loss is preventable. As such a widespread issue, NIOSH has been committed to preventing future hearing loss for workers by establishing recommended exposure limits (RELs) of 85 dB(A) for an 8-house time-weighed average (TWA). The Buy Quiet program was developed by NIOSH to encourage employers to reduce workplace noise levels by purchasing quieter models of tools and machinery. Additionally, a partnership with the National Hearing Conservation Association (NHCA) has resulted in the creation of the Safe-in-Sound Award to recognize excellence and innovation in the field of hearing loss prevention.

Occupational Cancer

Occupational cancer is cancer caused by occupational hazards. Several cancers have been directly tied to occupational hazards, including chimney sweeps' carcinoma, mesothelioma, and others.

Common Occupational Hazards Implicated in Cancer

Occupational exposure to chemicals, dusts, radiation, and certain industrial processes have been tied to occupational cancer. Exposure to cancer-causing chemicals, also called Carcinogens, may cause mutations that allow cells to grow out of control, causing cancer. Carcinogens in the workplace may include chemicals like anilines, chromates, dinitrotoluenes, arsenic and inorganic arsenic compounds, beryllium and beryllium compounds, cadmium compounds, and nickel compounds. Dusts that can cause cancer leather or wood dusts, asbestos, crystalline forms of silica, coal tar pitch volatiles, coke oven emissions, diesel exhaust and environmental tobacco smoke. sunlight; radon gas; and industrial, medical, or other exposure to ionizing radiation can all cause cancer in the workplace. Industrial processes associated with cancer include aluminum production; iron and steel founding; and underground mining with exposure to uranium or radon.

Other factors that play a role in cancer include:

- Personal characteristics such as age, sex, and race
- Family history of cancer
- Diet and personal habits such as cigarette smoking and alcohol consumption
- The presence of certain medical conditions or past medical treatments, including chemotherapy, radiation treatment, or some immune-system suppressing drugs.
- Exposure to cancer-causing agents in the environment (for example, sunlight, radon gas, air pollution, and infectious agents)

Occupational Cancers

Common cancers and their exposures and occupations include:

Cancer	Source	Examples of Occupations
Bladder	Benzidine, beta-naphthylamine, 4-aminobiphenyl, arsenic	Rubber, leather, paving, roofing, printing and textile industries; paint/dyeing products; chimney sweeping; machinists; hairdressers and barbers; truck drivers
Kidney	Cadmium, trichloroethylene, herbicides, wood dust	Painting; metalworking; petroleum, plastics, and textile industries
Larynx	Asbestos, wood dust, paint fumes	Metal working; petroleum, rubber, plastics, and textile industries
Leukemia	Formaldehyde, benzene, ethylene oxide, pesticides	Rubber manufacturing; oil refining; shoemaking
Liver	Arsenic, vinyl chloride, aflatoxins	Plastic manufacturing
Lung	Radon, secondhand smoke, asbestos, arsenic, cadmium, chromium compounds, diesel exhaust, sulfur mustard	Rubber manufacturing, paving, roofing, painting, chimney sweeping, iron and steel foundry work, welding
Lymphoma	Benzene, 1, 3-butadiene, ethylene oxide, herbicides, insecticides	Rubber manufacturing, painting, hairdresser or barber
Mesothelioma	Asbestos	Mining, railroad, automotive, plumbing, painting and construction industries; factory workers

Nasal cavity and sinus	Mustard gas, nickel dust, chromium dust, leather dust, wood dust, radium	Textile and baking industry, flour milling, nickel refining, furniture and cabinet builders, shoemaking
Skin	Arsenic, coal tars, paraffin, certain oils, sunlight	Chimney sweeping; outside jobs that involve a lot of sun exposure

Epidemiology

An estimated 48,000 cancers are diagnosed yearly in the US that come from occupational causes; this represents approximately 4-10% of total cancer in the United States. It is estimated that 19% of cancers globally are attributed to environmental exposures (including work-related exposures).

Prevention

Many occupational cancers are preventable. Personal protective gear, workplace controls, and worker education can prevent exposure to carcinogens in the workplace. Tobacco smoking has also been shown to increase the risk of work-related cancers; decreasing or abstaining from smoking can decrease cancer risk.

Agencies like the US Food and Drug Administration, Environmental Protection Agency, and Occupational Safety and Health Administration have developed safety standards and limits for chemical and radiation exposure.

Work Accident

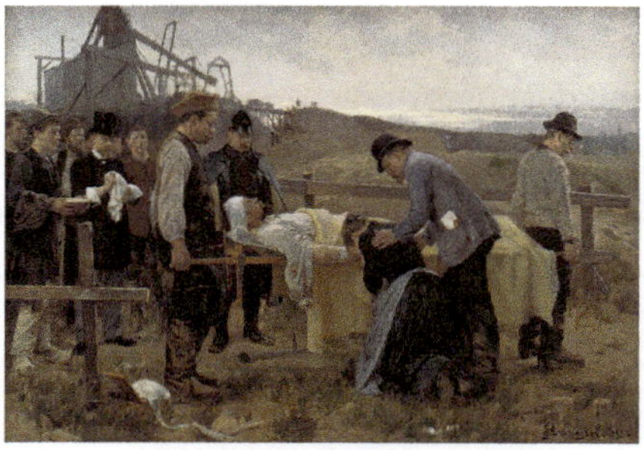

Erik Henningsen's painting *A wounded worker* from the National Gallery of Denmark

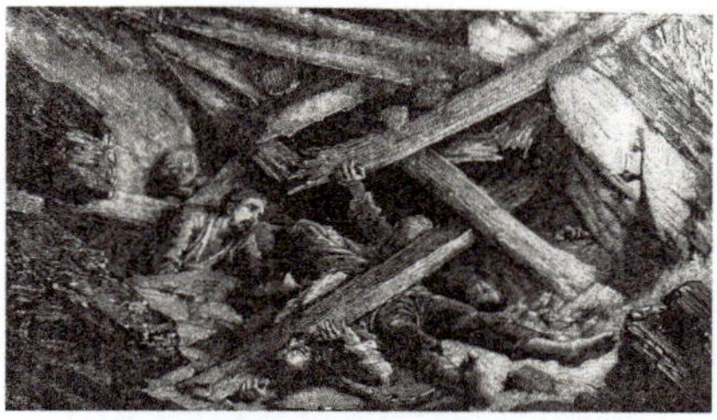

A 19th century work accident in a mine

A work accident, workplace accident, occupational accident, or accident at work is a "discrete occurrence in the course of work" leading to physical or mental occupational injury. According to the International Labour Organization (ILO), more than 337 million accidents happen on the job each year, resulting, together with occupational diseases, in more than 2.3 million deaths annually.

The phrase "in the course of work" can include work-related accidents happening off the company's premises, and can include accidents caused by third parties, according to Eurostat. The definition of work accident includes accidents occurring "while engaged in an economic activity, or at work, or carrying on the business of the employer" according to the ILO.

The phrase "physical or mental harm" means any injury, disease, or death. Occupational accidents differ from occupational diseases as accidents are unexpected and unplanned occurrences (e.g., mine collapse), while occupational diseases are "contracted as a result of an exposure over a period of time to risk factors arising from work activity" (e.g., miner's lung).

Incidents that fall within the definition of occupational accidents include cases of acute poisoning, attacks by humans and animals, insects etc., slips and falls on pavements or staircases, traffic collisions, and accidents on board means of transportation in the course of work, accidents in airports, stations and so on.

There is no consensus as to whether commuting accidents (i.e. accidents on the way to work and while returning home after work) should be considered to be work accidents. The ESAW methodology excludes them; the ILO includes them in its conventions concerning Health & Safety at work, although it lists them as a separate category of accidents; and some countries (e.g., Greece) do not distinguish them from other work accidents.

A fatal accident at work is defined as an accident which leads to the death of a victim. The time within which the death may occur varies among countries: In Netherlands an accident is registered as fatal if the victim dies during the same day that the accident happened, in Germany if death came within 30 days, while Belgium, France and Greece set no time limit.

Where the accidents involve multiple fatalities they are often referred to as industrial disasters.

Types

Although many workplace accidents have relatively minor repercussions, which could result in just a paper cut or scratch, others can have more serious – and potentially fatal – consequences.

For instance, there are some industries in which individuals are more exposed to occupational hazards than others, such as the construction trade. This had the highest rate of fatal injuries out of all other industry sections in 2011/12. During this period, falls accounted for 51% of construction injuries resulting in death, demonstrating that builders are more likely to fall from height than those who work in less dangerous locations, such as an office.

An independent watchdog – the Health and Safety Executive (HSE) – aims to reduce the number of work-related fatalities and injuries within Great Britain, publishing statistics that show the different – and most common – types of reported workplace injuries across a range of sectors.

For example, the HSE reported that, between 2011 and 2012, incidents such as falls from height, becoming trapped by a falling structure, and being struck by a vehicle or moving object, were the reasons for the majority of fatalities to British workers.

It was also revealed that slips, trips or falls were responsible for more than 50% of serious injuries to employees. Furthermore, the majority of incidents that resulted in employees taking more than three days off work – or affected their ability to perform their usual duties over this period – were caused by handling accidents.

Although some accidents at work can have minor effects, the HSE statistics revealed that more than 27 million working days were lost between 2011 and 2012 due to occupational illness or personal injury, proving that these incidents can have serious repercussions.

Causal Factors

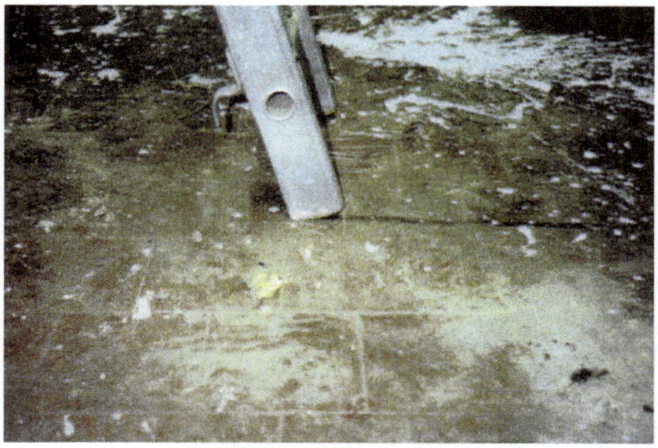

Skid mark from a faulty ladder.

Accidents arise from unsafe behavior and/or unsafe conditions. An important factor is the safety climate or safety culture of an organization. Safety culture concerns how workplace safety is managed, consisting of the shared attitudes, beliefs, perceptions, and values among employees. Faulty equipment can also cause serious personal injuries, a common example being accidents from faulty ladders. If the rubber feet are absent, the base of the aluminium stile can slip suddenly on a hard floor and the user fall.

Benefits of Prevention

Health and safety warning sign

According to the Health and Safety Executive, employers who implement suitable measures to prevent accidents in the workplace could reap a number of benefits. As well as reducing the number of injuries at work, managers could also:

- Be less likely to suffer legal action
- Acquire a better reputation amongst partners, investors, customers and suppliers
- Have employees who feel more motivated, demonstrating greater productivity
- Reduce costs
- Have reduced employee turnover and absence rates. It has been reported that over 2,000,000 working days each year are lost due to handling accidents and slips and trips alone.

Example

Harry Potter and the Deathly Hallows movie, year 2009, David Holmes, a stuntman, paralysed after getting blown by explosion, suffered impact to a wall .

Transformers:Dark of the Moon, year 2010, a stuntwoman suffered brain damage after her car was hit by a cable then crash to central barrier .

The Expendables 2, year 2011, Kun Lieu, stuntman, died because of accidental explosion during filming.

Resident Evil: The Final Chapter movie, year 2015, Olivia Jackson, stuntwoman, had her arm amputated after her motorbike crashed to a metal camera arm during high-speed chase .

Midnight Rider movie, 20 February 2014, camera assistant, Sarah Jones, died after getting hit by CSX freight train during filming

The Dark Knight movie, year 2007, cameraman Conway Wickliffe died when his car crashed to a tree while following a stunt car batmobile.

Steep video game, 18 July 2016, free-skier, Matilda Hargin née Rapaport died from an avalanche while filming an advertisement.

Occupational Exposure Limit

An occupational exposure limit is an upper limit on the acceptable concentration of a hazardous substance in workplace air for a particular material or class of materials. It is typically set by competent national authorities and enforced by legislation to protect occupational safety and health. It is an important tool in risk assessment and in the management of activities involving handling of dangerous substances. There are many dangerous substances for which there are no formal occupational exposure limits. In these cases, hazard banding or control banding strategies can be used to ensure safe handling.

Background

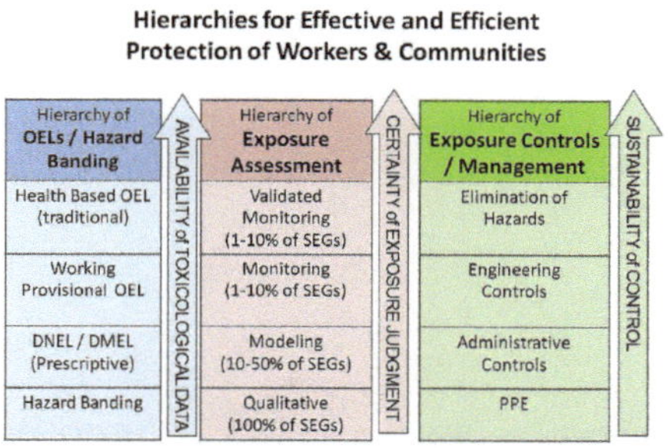

Simple representation of exposure risk assessment and management hierarchy based on available information

Occupational Exposure Limits (OELs) have been established for airborne workplace chemicals by multiple regulatory and authoritative organizations around the world for well over 60 years now. With the changing regulatory arena, shifting centers of manufacturing growth, and the move towards a more global view on occupational hygiene issues, it is important for the Occupational Hygiene profession to understand the current and growing issues impacting the continued viability of OEL's in our professional practice.

Although peer-reviewed health-based OELs are preferred for establishing safe levels of exposure or for implementing adequate controls to provide worker protection, the lack of publicly available OELs have led to other sources of safe levels to protect workers. Industrial or Occupational Hygienists are often on the front line of anticipating and recognizing the hazards of chemical exposure for workers, and must assess the risk of exposure through the use of OELs so that proper control strategies can be implemented to keep workers below the OEL values. In the absence of OELs however, there are a variety of tools that can and should be used to assess exposure potential of workers. The

"Hierarchy of OELs" provides a continuum of occupational exposure limit values that allow assessment of the risk of exposure in order to apply adequate controls.

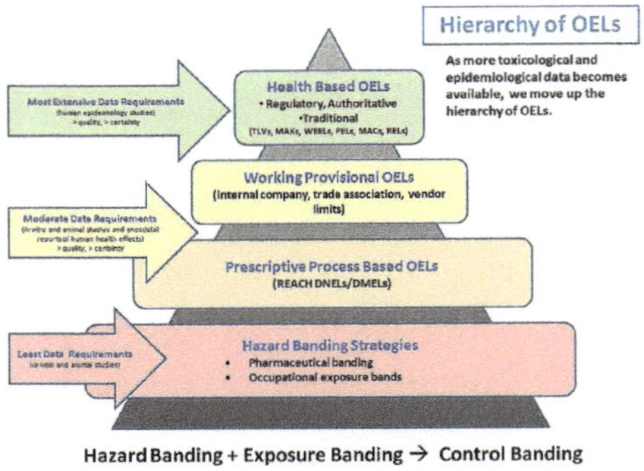

Hierarchy of occupational exposure limits (OELs)

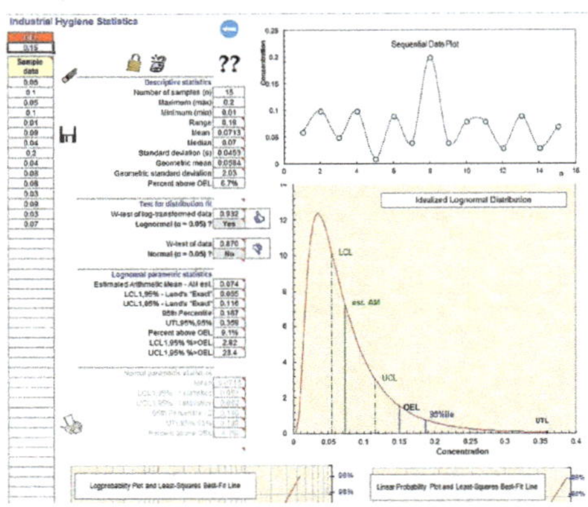

Illustration of statistical output from IHSTAT using air sampling data

Personal air sampling is routinely conducted on workers to determine whether exposures are acceptable or unacceptable. These samples are collected and analyzed using validated sampling and analytical methods. These methods are available from OSHA Technical Manual and NIOSH Manual of Analytical Methods Statistical tools are available to assess exposure monitoring data against OELs. The statistical tools are typically free but do require some previous knowledge with statistical concepts. A popular exposure data statistical tool called "IH STAT" is available from AIHA (American Industrial Hygiene Association). IHSTAT has 14 languages including English and is available for free.

Methods for performing occupational exposure assessments can be found in "A Strategy for Assessing and Managing Occupational Exposures, Third Edition Edited by Joselito S. Ignacio and William H. Bullock".

Types

- Permissible exposure limit, set by the U.S. Occupational Safety and Health Administration

- Recommended exposure limit, set by the U.S. National Institute for Occupational Safety and Health
- Indicative limit value, set by the European Union
- Threshold limit value, set by the American Conference of Governmental Industrial Hygienists
- Occupational exposure banding, a process that can be used when not enough data are available to determine quantiative exposure limits

Occupational Safety and Health

Occupational safety and health (OSH), also commonly referred to as occupational health and safety (OHS), occupational health, or workplace health and safety (WHS), is a multidisciplinary field concerned with the safety, health, and welfare of people at work. These terms of course also refer to the goals of this field, so their use in the sense of this article was originally an abbreviation of *occupational safety and health program/department* etc.

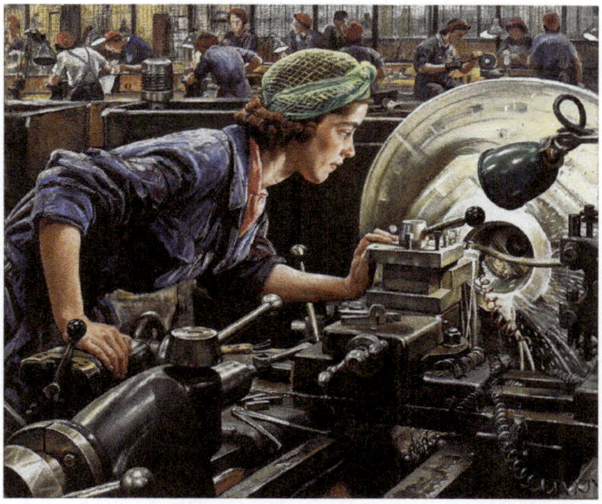

This painting depicts a woman examining her work on a lathe at a factory in Britain during World War II. Her eyes are not protected. Today, such practice would not be permitted in most industrialized countries that adhere to occupational health and safety standards for workers. In many countries however, such standards are still either weak or nonexistent.

The goals of occupational safety and health programs include to foster a safe and healthy work environment. OSH may also protect co-workers, family members, employers, customers, and many others who might be affected by the workplace environment. In the United States, the term occupational health and safety is referred to as occupational health and occupational and non-occupational safety and includes safety for activities outside of work.

In common-law jurisdictions, employers have a common law duty to take reasonable care of the safety of their employees. Statute law may in addition impose other general duties, introduce specific duties, and create government bodies with powers to regulate workplace safety issues: details of this vary from jurisdiction to jurisdiction.

Definition

As defined by the World Health Organization (WHO) "occupational health deals with all aspects of health and safety in the workplace and has a strong focus on primary prevention of hazards." Health has been defined as "a state of complete physical, mental and social well-being and not merely the absence of disease or infirmity." Occupational health is a multidisciplinary field of healthcare concerned with enabling an individual to undertake their occupation, in the way that causes least harm to their health. Health has been defined as It contrasts, for example, with the promotion of health and safety at work, which is concerned with preventing harm from any incidental hazards, arising in the workplace.

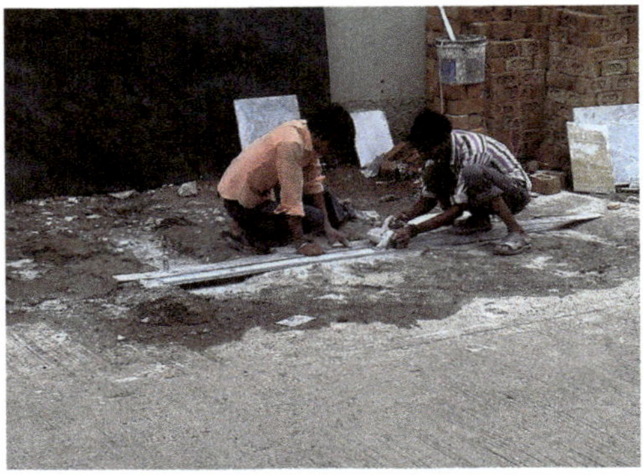

Workers cutting marble without any protective gear, Indore, India

Since 1950, the International Labour Organization (ILO) and the World Health Organization (WHO) have shared a common definition of occupational health. It was adopted by the Joint ILO/WHO Committee on Occupational Health at its first session in 1950 and revised at its twelfth session in 1995. The definition reads:

"The main focus in occupational health is on three different objectives: (i) the maintenance and promotion of workers' health and working capacity; (ii) the improvement of working environment and work to become conducive to safety and health and (iii) development of work organizations and working cultures in a direction which supports health and safety at work and in doing so also promotes a positive social climate and smooth operation and may enhance productivity of the undertakings. The concept of working culture is intended in this context to mean a reflection of the essential value systems adopted by the undertaking concerned. Such a culture is reflected in practice in the managerial systems, personnel policy, principles for participation, training policies and quality management of the undertaking."

—Joint ILO/WHO Committee on Occupational Health

Those in the field of occupational health come from a wide range of disciplines and professions including medicine, psychology, epidemiology, physiotherapy and rehabilitation, occupational therapy, occupational medicine, human factors and ergonomics, and many others. Professionals advise on a broad range of occupational health matters. These include how to avoid particular pre-existing conditions causing a problem in the occupation, correct posture for the work, frequency of rest breaks, preventative action that can be undertaken, and so forth.

"Occupational health should aim at: the promotion and maintenance of the highest degree of physical, mental and social well-being of workers in all occupations; the prevention amongst workers of departures from health caused by their working conditions; the protection of workers in their employment from risks resulting from factors adverse to health; the placing and maintenance of the worker in an occupational environment adapted to his physiological and psychological capabilities; and, to summarize, the adaptation of work to man and of each man to his job.

History

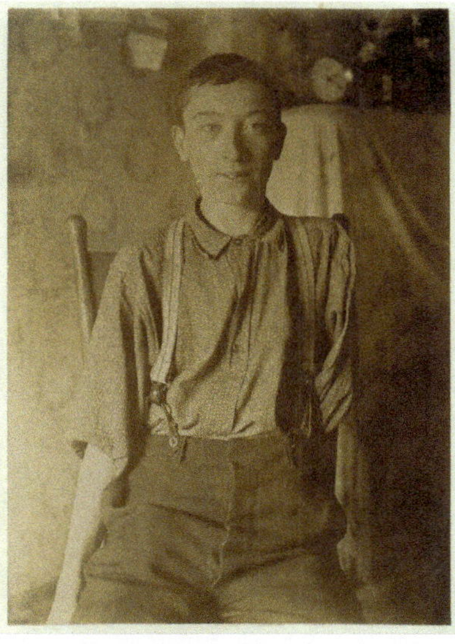

Harry McShane, age 16, 1908. Pulled into machinery in a factory in Cincinnati and had his arm ripped off at the shoulder and his leg broken without any compensation.

The research and regulation of occupational safety and health are a relatively recent phenomenon. As labor movements arose in response to worker concerns in the wake of the industrial revolution, worker's health entered consideration as a labor-related issue.

In the United Kingdom, the Factory Acts of the early nineteenth century (from 1802 onwards) arose out of concerns about the poor health of children working in cotton mills: the Act of 1833 created a dedicated professional Factory Inspectorate. The initial remit of the Inspectorate was to police restrictions on the working hours in the textile industry of children and young persons (introduced to prevent chronic overwork, identified as leading directly to ill-health and deformation, and indirectly to a high accident rate). However, on the urging of the Factory Inspectorate, a further Act in 1844 giving similar restrictions on working hours for women in the textile industry introduced a requirement for machinery guarding (but only in the textile industry, and only in areas that might be accessed by women or children).

In 1840 a Royal Commission published its findings on the state of conditions for the workers of the mining industry that documented the appallingly dangerous environment that they had to work in and the high frequency of accidents. The commission sparked public outrage which resulted in the Mines Act of 1842. The act set up an inspectorate for mines and collieries which resulted in many prosecutions and safety improvements, and by 1850, inspectors were able to enter and inspect premises at their discretion.

Otto von Bismarck inaugurated the first social insurance legislation in 1883 and the first worker's compensation law in 1884 – the first of their kind in the Western world. Similar acts followed in other countries, partly in response to labor unrest.

Workplace Hazards

Although work provides many economic and other benefits, a wide array of workplace hazards also present risks to the health and safety of people at work. These include but are not limited to, "chemicals, biological agents, physical factors, adverse ergonomic conditions, allergens, a complex network of safety risks," and a broad range of psychosocial risk factors. Personal protective equipment can help protect against many of these hazards.

Physical hazards affect many people in the workplace. Occupational hearing loss is the most common work-related injury in the United States, with 22 million workers exposed to hazardous noise levels at work and an estimated $242 million spent annually on worker's compensation for hearing loss disability. Falls are also a common cause of occupational injuries and fatalities, especially in construction, extraction, transportation, healthcare, and building cleaning and maintenance. Machines have moving parts, sharp edges, hot surfaces and other hazards with the potential to crush, burn, cut, shear, stab or otherwise strike or wound workers if used unsafely.

Biological hazards (biohazards) include infectious microorganisms such as viruses and toxins produced by those organisms such as anthrax. Biohazards affect workers in many industries; influenza, for example, affects a broad population of workers. Outdoor workers, including farmers, landscapers, and construction workers, risk exposure to numerous biohazards, including animal bites and stings, urushiol from poisonous plants, and diseases transmitted through animals such as the West Nile virus and Lyme disease. Health care workers, including veterinary health workers, risk exposure to blood-borne pathogens and various infectious diseases, especially those that are emerging.

Dangerous chemicals can pose a chemical hazard in the workplace. There are many classifications of hazardous chemicals, including neurotoxins, immune agents, dermatologic agents, carcinogens, reproductive toxins, systemic toxins, asthmagens, pneumoconiotic agents, and sensitizers. Authorities such as regulatory agencies set occupational exposure limits to mitigate the risk of chemical hazards. An international effort is investigating the health effects of mixtures of chemicals. There is some evidence that certain chemicals are harmful at lower levels when mixed with one or more other chemicals. This may be particularly important in causing cancer.

Psychosocial hazards include risks to the mental and emotional well-being of workers, such as feelings of job insecurity, long work hours, and poor work-life balance. A recent Cochrane review - using moderate quality evidence - related that the addition of work-directed interventions for depressed workers receiving clinical interventions reduces the number of lost work days as compared to clinical interventions alone. This review also demonstrated that the addition of cognitive behavioral therapy to primary or occupational care and the addition of a "structured telephone outreach and care management program" to usual care are both effective at reducing sick leave days.

By Industry

Specific occupational safety and health risk factors vary depending on the specific sector and industry. Construction workers might be particularly at risk of falls, for instance, whereas fishermen might be particularly at risk of drowning. The United States Bureau of Labor Statistics identifies the fishing, aviation, lumber, metalworking, agriculture, mining and transportation industries as among some of the more dangerous for workers. Similarly psychosocial risks such as workplace violence are more pronounced for certain occupational groups such as health care employees, police, correctional officers and teachers.

Construction

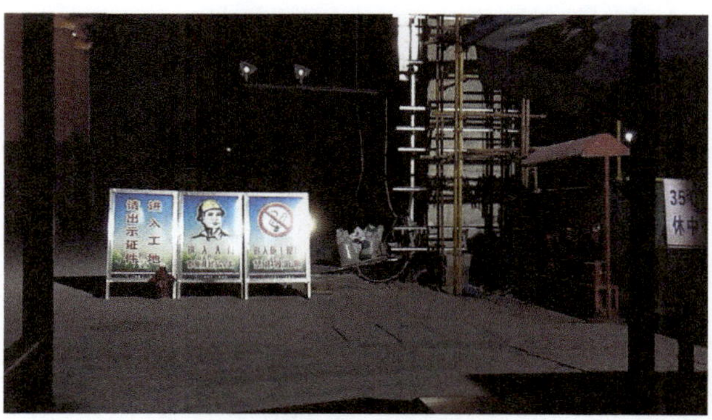

Workplace safety notices at the entrance of a Chinese construction site.

Construction is one of the most dangerous occupations in the world, incurring more occupational fatalities than any other sector in both the United States and in the European Union. In 2009, the fatal occupational injury rate among construction workers in the United States was nearly three times that for all workers. Falls are one of the most common causes of fatal and non-fatal injuries among construction workers. Proper safety equipment such as harnesses and guardrails and procedures such as securing ladders and inspecting scaffolding can curtail the risk of occupational injuries in the construction industry. Due to the fact that accidents may have disastrous consequences for employees as well as organizations, it is of utmost importance to ensure health and safety of workers and compliance with HSE construction requirements. Health and safety legislation in the construction industry involves many rules and regulations. For example, the role of the Construction Design Management (CDM) Coordinator as a requirement has been aimed at improving health and safety on-site.

The 2010 National Health Interview Survey Occupational Health Supplement (NHIS-OHS) identified work organization factors and occupational psychosocial and chemical/physical exposures which may increase some health risks. Among all U.S. workers in the construction sector, 44% had non-standard work arrangements (were not regular permanent employees) compared to 19% of all U.S. workers, 15% had temporary employment compared to 7% of all U.S. workers, and 55% experienced job insecurity compared to 32% of all U.S. workers. Prevalence rates for exposure to physical/chemical hazards were especially high for the construction sector. Among nonsmoking workers, 24% of construction workers were exposed to secondhand smoke while only 10% of all U.S. workers were exposed. Other physical/chemical hazards with high prevalence rates in the construction industry were frequently working outdoors (73%) and frequent exposure to vapors, gas, dust, or fumes (51%).

Agriculture

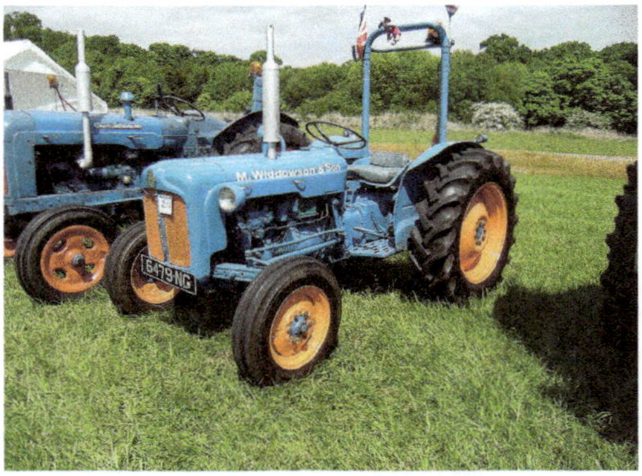

Rollover protection bar on a Fordson tractor.

Agriculture workers are often at risk of work-related injuries, lung disease, noise-induced hearing loss, skin disease, as well as certain cancers related to chemical use or prolonged sun exposure. On industrialized farms, injuries frequently involve the use of agricultural machinery. The most common cause of fatal agricultural injuries in the United States is tractor rollovers, which can be prevented by the use of roll over protection structures which limit the risk of injury in case a tractor rolls over. Pesticides and other chemicals used in farming can also be hazardous to worker health, and workers exposed to pesticides may experience illnesses or birth defects. As an industry in which families, including children, commonly work alongside their families, agriculture is a common source of occupational injuries and illnesses among younger workers. Common causes of fatal injuries among young farm worker include drowning, machinery and motor vehicle-related accidents.

The 2010 NHIS-OHS found elevated prevalence rates of several occupational exposures in the agriculture, forestry, and fishing sector which may negatively impact health. These workers often worked long hours. The prevalence rate of working more than 48 hours a week among workers employed in these industries was 37%, and 24% worked more than 60 hours a week. Of all workers in these industries, 85% frequently worked outdoors compared to 25% of all U.S. workers. Additionally, 53% were frequently exposed to vapors, gas, dust, or fumes, compared to 25% of all U.S. workers.

Service Sector

As the number of service sector jobs has risen in developed countries, more and more jobs have become sedentary, presenting a different array of health problems than those associated with manufacturing and the primary sector. Contemporary problems such as the growing rate of obesity and issues relating to occupational stress, workplace bullying, and overwork in many countries have further complicated the interaction between work and health.

According to data from the 2010 NHIS-OHS, hazardous physical/chemical exposures in the service sector were lower than national averages. On the other hand, potentially harmful work organization characteristics and psychosocial workplace exposures were relatively common in this sector. Among all workers in the service industry, 30% experienced job insecurity in 2010, 27% worked non-standard shifts (not a regular day shift), 21% had non-standard work arrangements (were not regular permanent employees).

Due to the manual labour involved and on a per employee basis, the US Postal Service, UPS and Fedex are the 4th, 5th and 7th most dangerous companies to work for in the US.

Mining and Oil & Gas Extraction

According to data from the 2010 NHIS-OHS, workers employed in mining and oil and gas extraction industries had high prevalence rates of exposure to potentially harmful work organization characteristics and hazardous chemicals. Many of these workers worked long hours: 50% worked more than 48 hours a week and 25% worked more than 60 hours a week in 2010. Additionally, 42% worked non-standard shifts (not a regular day shift). These workers also had high prevalence of exposure to physical/chemical hazards. In 2010, 39% had frequent skin contact with chemicals. Among nonsmoking workers, 28% of those in mining and oil and gas extraction industries had frequent exposure to secondhand smoke at work. About two-thirds were frequently exposed to vapors, gas, dust, or fumes at work.

Healthcare and Social Assistance

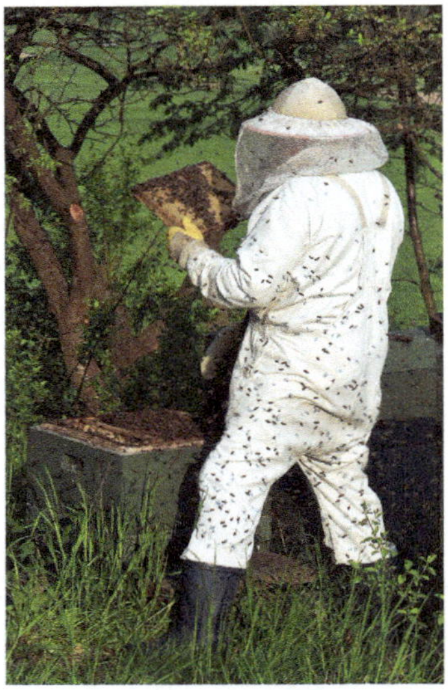

Beekeepers often wear protective clothing, for OHS reasons

Healthcare workers are exposed to many hazards that can adversely affect their health and well-being. Long hours, changing shifts, physically demanding tasks, violence, and exposures to infectious diseases and harmful chemicals are examples of hazards that put these workers at risk for illness and injury.

According to the Bureau of Labor statistics, U.S. hospitals recorded 253,700 work-related injuries and illnesses in 2011, which is 6.8 work-related injuries and illnesses for every 100 full-time employees. The injury and illness rate in hospitals is higher than the rates in construction and manufacturing – two industries that are traditionally thought to be relatively hazardous.

The Occupational Health Safety Network (OHSN) is a secure electronic surveillance system developed by the National Institute for Occupational Safety and Health (NIOSH) to address health and safety risks among health care personnel. OHSN uses existing data to characterize risk of injury and illness among health care workers. Hospitals and other healthcare facilities can upload the occupational injury data they already collect to the secure database for analysis and benchmarking with other de-identified facilities. NIOSH works with OHSN participants in identifying and implementing timely and targeted interventions. OHSN modules currently focus on three high risk and preventable events that can lead to injuries or musculoskeletal disorders among healthcare personnel: musculoskeletal injuries from patient handling activities; slips, trips, and falls; and workplace violence. OHSN enrollment is open to all healthcare facilities.

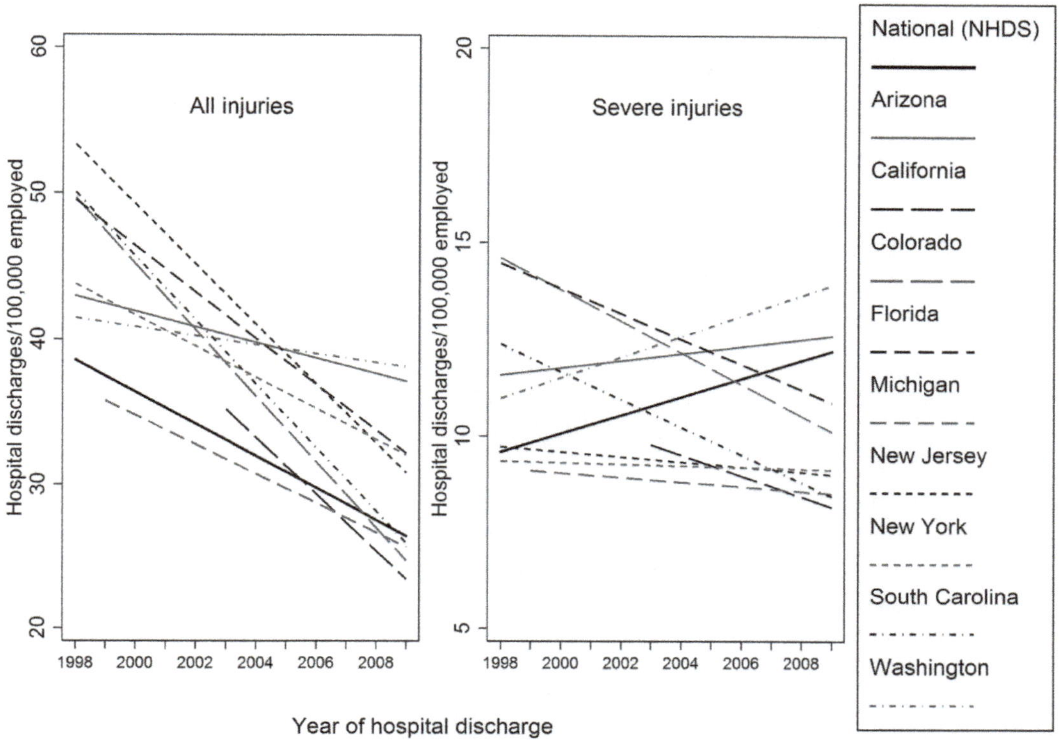

Workplace Fatality and Injury Statistics

United States

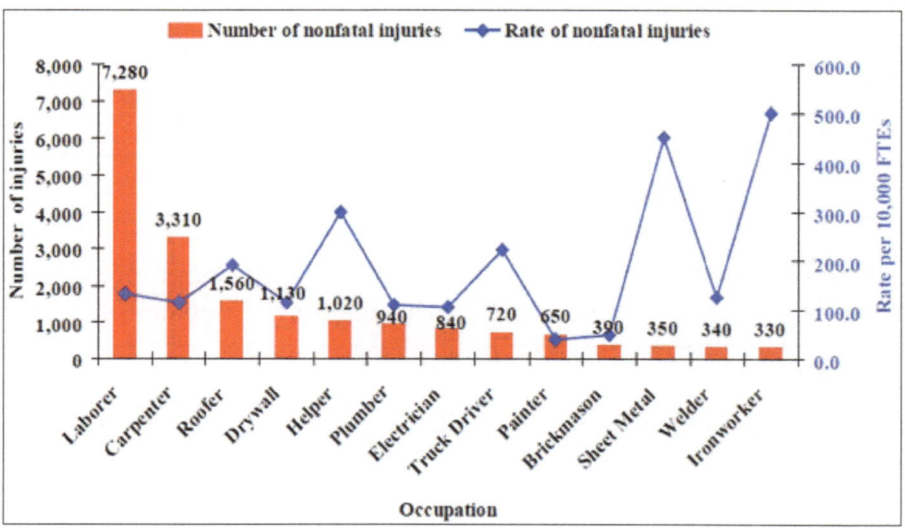

The Bureau of Labor Statistics of the United States Department of Labor compiles information about workplace fatalities and non-fatal injuries in the United States. In 1970, an estimated 14,000 workers were killed on the job – by 2010, the workforce had doubled, but workplace deaths were down to about 4,500. Between 1913 and 2013, workplace fatalities dropped by approximately 80%.

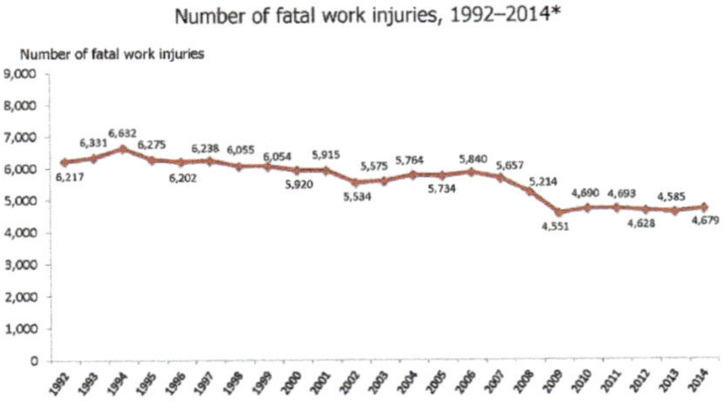

Number of occupational fatal work injuries in the U.S. from 1992 until 2014. Note, 2001 statistics do not include death related to the September 11 terrorist attacks.

The Bureau also compiles information about the most dangerous jobs. According to the census of occupational injuries 4,679 people died on the job in 2014.In 2015, a decline in nonfatal workplace injuries and illnesses was observed, with private industry employers reporting approximately 2.9 million incidents, nearly 48,000 fewer cases than in 2014.

Job	Fatalities	Fatalities per 100,000 employees
Fishermen	22	80.8
Pilots	81	63.2
Timber cutter	77	109.5
Structural metal workers	15	25.2
Waste collectors	27	35.8
Farmers and ranchers	263	26.0
Power-line workers	25	19.2
Construction workers and miners	130	17.9
Roofers	81	46.2
Truck drivers and other drivers	835	23.4
All occupations	**4,679**	**3.3**

Cause of injury and illness	2014 rate per 10,000 full-time employees
Contact with objects	23.8
Fall to lower level	5.4
Fall on same level	18.8
Slips or trips without fall	4.4
Over-exertion in lifting/lowering	11.0
Repetitive motion	2.7
Exposure to harmful substances or environments	4.3

Cause of injury and illness	2014 rate per 10,000 full-time employees
Transportation incidents	5.8
Fires and explosions	0.2
Violence and other injuries by person or animal	6.8
Total	**107.1**

Musculoskeletal injuries accounted for 32% of all employer-reported injuries and illnesses in 2014.

European Union

In most countries males comprise the vast majority of workplace fatalities. In the EU as a whole, 94% of death were of males. In the UK the disparity was even greater with males comprising 97.4% of workplace deaths. In the UK there were 171 fatal injuries at work in financial year 2011–2012, compared with 651 in calendar year 1974; the fatal injury rate declined over that period from 2.9 fatalities per 100,000 workers to 0.6 per 100,000 workers

Management Systems

International

In 2001, the International Labour Organization (ILO) published ILO-OSH 2001, also titled "Guidelines a on occupational safety and health management systems" to assist organizations with introducing OSH management systems. These guidelines encourage continual improvement in employee health and safety, achieved via a constant process of policy, organization, planning & implementation, evaluation, and action for improvement, all supported by constant auditing to determine the success of OSH actions.

The ILO management system was created to assist employers to keep pace with rapidly shifting and competitive industrial environments. The ILO recognizes that national legislation is essential, but sometimes insufficient on its own to address the challenges faced by industry, and therefore elected to ensure free and open distribution of administrative tools in the form of occupational health and safety management system guidance for everyone. This open access forum is intended to provide the tools for industry to create safe and healthy working environments and foster positive safety cultures within the organizations.

OHSAS 18000 is an international occupational health and safety management system specification developed by the London-based BSI Group, a multinational business chiefly concerned with the production and distribution of standards related services. OHSAS 18000 comprises two parts, OHSAS 18001 and 18002 and embraces a number of other publications. OHSAS 18000 is the internationally recognized assessment specification for occupational health and safety management systems. It was developed by a selection of leading trade bodies, international standards and certification bodies to address a gap where no third-party certifiable international standard exists. This internationally recognized specification for occupational health and safety management system operates on the basis of policy, planning, implementation and operation, checking and corrective action, management review, and continual improvement.

The British Standards – Occupational Health and Safety management Systems Requirements Standard BS OHSAS 18001 was developed within the framework of the ISO standards series. Allowing it to integrate better into the larger system of ISO certifications. ISO 9001 Quality Management Systems and ISO 14001 Environmental Management System can work in tandem with BS OHSAS 18001/18002 to complement each other and form a better overall system. Each component of the system is specific, auditable, and accreditable by a third party after review.

Also Standards Australia and the Association Française de Normalisation (AFNOR) in France have developed occupational safety and health management standards.

United Kingdom

Guidance note HSG65: Successful Health and Safety Management, published by the British non-departmental public body Health and Safety Executive, was substantially re-written 2013. It now promotes the Plan Do Check Act approach to health and safety management, sharing similarities with BS OHSAS 18001. This achieved a balance between the original systems-based approach, and the more modern behavioural approach to safety management.

National Legislation and Public Organizations

Occupational safety and health practice vary among nations with different approaches to legislation, regulation, enforcement, and incentives for compliance. In the EU, for example, some member states promote OSH by providing public monies as subsidies, grants or financing, while others have created tax system incentives for OSH investments. A third group of EU member states has experimented with using workplace accident insurance premium discounts for companies or organisations with strong OSH records.

Australia

In Australia, the Commonwealth, four of the six states and both territories have enacted and administer harmonised Work Health and Safety Legislation in accordance with the *Intergovernmental Agreement for Regulatory and Operational Reform in Occupational Health and Safety*. Each of these jurisdictions has enacted Work Health & Safety legislation and regulations based on the Commonwealth Work Health and Safety Act 2011 and common Codes of Practice developed by Safe Work Australia. Some jurisdictions have also included mine safety under the model approach, however, most have retained separate legislation for the time being. Western Australia intends to adopt a moderated version of the model approach and Victoria has retained its own regime, although the Model WHS laws themselves drew heavily on the Victoria approach.

Canada

In Canada, workers are covered by provincial or federal labour codes depending on the sector in which they work. Workers covered by federal legislation (including those in mining, transportation, and federal employment) are covered by the Canada Labour Code; all other workers are covered by the health and safety legislation of the province in which they work. The Canadian Centre for Occupational Health and Safety (CCOHS), an agency of the Government of Canada, was created in 1966 by an Act of Parliament. The act was based on the belief that all Canadians had "...a fundamental right to a healthy and safe working environment." CCOHS is mandated to promote safe and healthy workplaces to help prevent work-related injuries and illnesses. The CCOHS maintains a useful (partial) list of OSH regulations for Canada and its provinces.

European Union

Number of full-time OSH inspectors per 100,000 full-time employees	
Italy	17.7
Finland	17.5
Denmark	11.9
United Kingdom	11.1
Norway	10.6
Sweden	10
Belgium	5.3
Netherlands	4.8
Ireland	4.5
Greece	4.1
France	3.5
Spain	2.1

In the European Union, member states have enforcing authorities to ensure that the basic legal requirements relating to occupational health and safety are met. In many EU countries, there is strong cooperation between employer and worker organisations (e.g. unions) to ensure good OSH performance as it is recognized this has benefits for both the worker (through maintenance of health) and the enterprise (through improved productivity and quality). In 1996, the European Agency for Safety and Health at Work was founded.

Member states of the European Union have all transposed into their national legislation a series of directives that establish minimum standards on occupational health and safety. These directives (of which there are about 20 on a variety of topics) follow a similar structure requiring the employer to assess the workplace risks and put in place preventive measures based on a hierarchy of control. This hierarchy starts with elimination of the hazard and ends with personal protective equipment.

However, certain EU member states admit to having lacking quality control in occupational safety services, to situations in which risk analysis takes place without any on-site workplace visits and to insufficient implementation of certain EU OSH directives. Based on this, it is hardly surprising that the total societal costs of work-related health problems and accidents vary from 2.6% to 3.8% of GNP between the EU member states.

Denmark

In Denmark, occupational safety and health is regulated by the Danish Act on Working Environment and cooperation at the workplace. The Danish Working Environment Authority carries out inspections of companies, draws up more detailed rules on health and safety at work and provides information on health and safety at work. The result of each inspection is made public on the web pages of the Danish Working Environment Authority so that the general public, current and prospective employees, customers and other stakeholders can inform themselves about whether a given organization has passed the inspection, should they wish to do so.

Spain

In Spain, occupational safety and health is regulated by the Spanish Act on Prevention of Labour Risks. The Ministry of Employment and Social Security is the authority responsible for issues relating to labour environment. The National Institute for Labour Safety and Hygiene is the technical public Organization specialized in occupational safety and health.

Sweden

In Sweden, occupational safety and health is regulated by the Work Environment Act. The Swedish Work Environment Authority is the government agency responsible for issues relating to the working environment. The agency should work to disseminate information and furnish advice on OSH, has a mandate to carry out inspections, and a right to issue stipulations and injunctions to any non-compliant employer.

United Kingdom

In the UK, health and safety legislation is drawn up and enforced by the Health and Safety Executive and local authorities (the local council) under the Health and Safety at Work etc. Act 1974 (HASAWA). HASAWA introduced (section 2) a general duty on an employer to ensure, so far as is reasonably practicable, the health, safety and welfare at work of all his employees; with the intention of giving a legal framework supporting 'codes of practice' not in themselves having legal force but establishing a strong presumption as to what was reasonably practicable (deviations from them could be justified by appropriate risk assessment). The previous reliance on detailed prescriptive rule-setting was seen as having failed to respond rapidly enough to technological change, leaving new technologies potentially un-regulated or inappropriately regulated. HSE has continued to make some regulations giving absolute duties (where something must be done with no 'reasonable practicability' test) but in the UK the regulatory trend is away from prescriptive rules, and towards 'goal setting' and risk assessment. Recent major changes to the laws governing asbestos and fire safety management embrace the concept of risk assessment. The other key aspect of the UK legislation is a statutory mechanism for worker involvement through elected health and safety representatives and health and safety committees. This followed a similar approach in Scandinavia, and that approach has since been adopted in Australia, Canada, New Zealand and Malaysia, for example.

For the UK, the government organisation dealing with occupational health has been the Employment Medical Advisory Service but in 2014 a new occupational health organisation - the Health and Work Service - was created to provide advice and assistance to employers in order to get back to work employees on long-term sick-leave. The service, funded by government, will offer medical assessments and treatment plans, on a voluntary basis, to people on long-term absence from their employer; in return, the government will no longer foot the bill for Statutory Sick Pay provided by the employer to the individual.

India

In India, the Labour Ministry formulates national policies on occupational safety and health in factories and docks with advice and assistance from Directorate General of Factory Advice Service and Labour Institutes (DGFASLI), and enforces its Policies through inspectorates of factories and inspectorates of dock safety. DGFASLI is the technical arm of the Ministry of Labour & Employment, Government of India and advises the factories on various problems concerning safety, health, efficiency and well - being of the persons at work places. The DGFASLI provides technical support in formulating rules, conducting occupational safety surveys and also for conducting occupational safety training programs.

Malaysia

In Malaysia, the Department of Occupational Safety and Health (DOSH) under the Ministry of Human Resource is responsible to ensure that the safety, health and welfare of workers in both the public and private sector is upheld. DOSH is responsible to enforce the Factories and Machinery Act 1967 and the Occupational Safety and Health Act 1994.

People's Republic of China

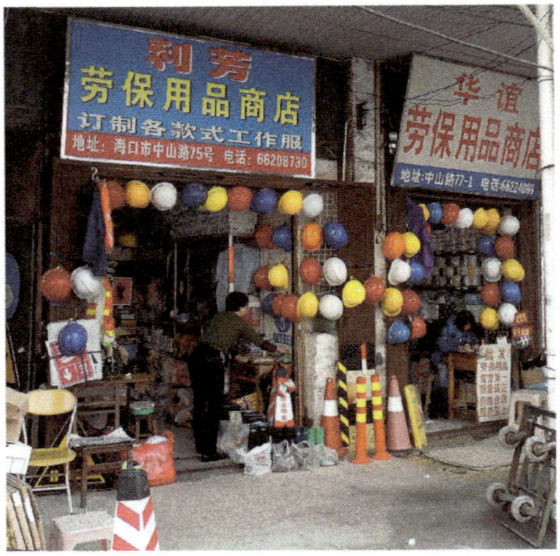

Hardware stores in China specializing in safety equipment

In the People's Republic of China, the Ministry of Health is responsible for occupational disease prevention and the State Administration of Work Safety for safety issues at work. On the provincial and municipal level, there are Health Supervisions for occupational health and local bureaus of Work Safety for safety. The "Occupational Disease Control Act of PRC" came into force on May 1, 2002. and Work safety Act of PRC on November 1, 2002. The Occupational Disease Control Act is under revision. The prevention of occupational disease is still in its initial stage compared with industrialised countries such as the US or UK.

Singapore

In Singapore, the Ministry of Manpower operates various checks and campaigns against unsafe work practices, such as when working at height, operating cranes and in traffic management. Examples include Operation Cormorant and the Falls Prevention Campaign.

South Africa

In South Africa the Department of Labour is responsible for occupational health and safety inspection and enforcement in commerce and industry apart from mining and energy production, where the Department of Mineral Resources is responsible.

The main statutory legislation on Health and Safety in the jurisdiction of the Department of Labour is *Act No. 85 of 1993: Occupational Health and Safety Act as amended by Occupational Health and Safety Amendment Act, No. 181 Of 1993.*

Regulations to the OHS Act include:

- *General Administrative Regulations, 2003*

- *Certificate of Competency Regulations, 1990*
- *Construction Regulations, 2014*
- *Diving Regulations 2009*
- *Driven Machinery Regulations, 1988*
- *Environmental Regulations for Workplaces, 1987*
- *General Machinery regulations, 1988*
- *General Safety Regulations, 1986*
- *Noise induced hearing loss regulations, 2003*
- *Pressure Equipment Regulations, 2004*

Taiwan

In Taiwan, the Occupational Safety and Health Administration of the Ministry of Labor is in charge of occupational safety and health. The matter is governed under the Occupational Safety and Health Act.

2007, official release the document TOSHMS (Taiwan Occupational Safety and Health Management System),which defined the basic rule about occupational safety standard.

United States

In the United States, President Richard Nixon signed the Occupational Safety and Health Act into law on December 29, 1970. The act created the three agencies that administer it. They include the Occupational Safety and Health Administration, National Institute for Occupational Safety and Health, and the Occupational Safety and Health Review Commission. The act authorized the Occupational Safety and Health Administration (OSHA) to regulate private employers in the 50 states, the District of Columbia, and territories. The Act establishing it includes a general duty clause requiring an employer to comply with the Act and regulations derived from it, and to provide employees with "employment and a place of employment which are free from recognized hazards that are causing or are likely to cause death or serious physical harm to his employees."

OSHA was established in 1971 under the Department of Labor. It has headquarters in Washington, DC and ten regional offices, further broken down into districts, each organized into three sections; compliance, training, and assistance. Its stated mission is *to assure safe and healthful working conditions for working men and women by setting and enforcing standards and by providing training, outreach, education and assistance*. The original plan was for OSHA to oversee 50 state plans with OSHA funding 50% of each plan. Unfortunately it has not worked out that way. There are currently 26 approved state plans (4 cover only public employees) and no other states want to participate. OSHA manages the plan in the states not participating.

OSHA develops safety standards in the Code of Federal Regulation and enforces those safety standards through compliance inspections conducted by Compliance Officers; enforcement resources are focussed on high-hazard industries. Worksites may apply to enter OSHA's Voluntary Protection Program (VPP); a successful application leads to an on-site inspection ; if this is passed the site gains VPP status and OSHA no longer inspect it annually nor (normally) visit it unless there is a fatal accident or an employee complaint until VPP revalidation (after 3–5 years)(VPP sites have injury and illness rates less than half the average for their industry).

It has 73 specialists in local offices to provide tailored information and training to employers and employees at little or no cost Similarly OSHA produces a range of publications, provides advice to employers and funds consultation services available for small businesses.

OSHA's Alliance Program enables groups committed to worker safety and health to work with it to develop compliance assistance tools and resources, share information with workers and employers, and educate them about their rights and responsibilities. OSHA also has a Strategic Partnership Program that zeros in on specific hazards or specific geographic areas. OSHA manages Susan B. Harwood grants to nonprofit companies to train workers and employers to recognize, avoid, and prevent safety and health hazards in the workplace. Grants focus on small business, hard-to-reach workers and high-hazard industries.

The National Institute for Occupational Safety and Health, created under the same act, works closely with OSHA and provides the research behind many of OSHA's regulations and standards.

Professional Roles and Responsibilities

The roles and responsibilities of OSH professionals vary regionally, but may include evaluating working environments, developing, endorsing and encouraging measures that might prevent injuries and illnesses, providing OSH information to employers, employees, and the public, providing medical examinations, and assessing the success of worker health programs.

Europe

In Norway, the main required tasks of an occupational health and safety practitioner include the following:

- Systematic evaluations of the working environment
- Endorsing preventative measures which eliminate causes of illnesses in the workplace

- Providing information on the subject of employees' health
- Providing information on occupational hygiene, ergonomics, and environmental and safety risks in the workplace

In the Netherlands, the required tasks for health and safety staff are only summarily defined and include the following:

- Providing voluntary medical examinations
- Providing a consulting room on the work environment to the workers
- Providing health assessments (if needed for the job concerned)

'The main influence of the Dutch law on the job of the safety professional is through the requirement on each employer to use the services of a certified working conditions service to advise them on health and safety'. A 'certified service' must employ sufficient numbers of four types of certified experts to cover the risks in the organisations which use the service:

- A safety professional
- An occupational hygienist
- An occupational physician
- A work and organisation specialist.

In 2004, 37% of health and safety practitioners in Norway and 14% in the Netherlands had an MSc; 44% had a BSc in Norway and 63% in the Netherlands; and 19% had training as an OSH technician in Norway and 23% in the Netherlands.

US

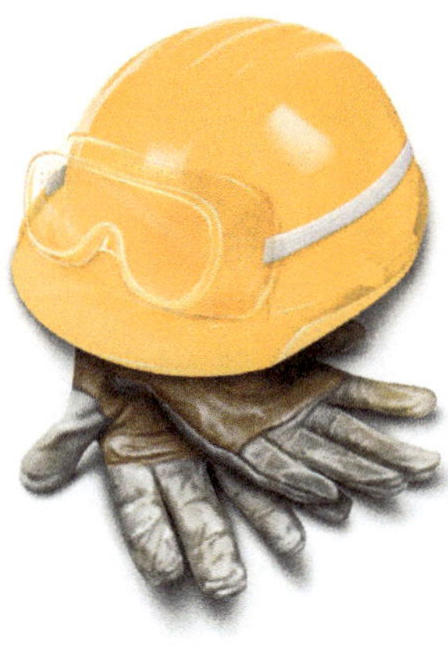

Leather craftsman gloves, safety goggles, and a properly fitted hardhat are crucial for proper safety in a construction environment.

The main tasks undertaken by the OHS practitioner in the US include:

- Develop processes, procedures, criteria, requirements, and methods to attain the best possible management of the hazards and exposures that can cause injury to people, and damage property, or the environment;
- Apply good business practices and economic principles for efficient use of resources to add to the importance of the safety processes;
- Promote other members of the company to contribute by exchanging ideas and other different approaches to make sure that every one in the corporation possess OHS knowledge and have functional roles in the development and execution of safety procedures;
- Assess services, outcomes, methods, equipment, workstations, and procedures by using qualitative and quantitative methods to recognise the hazards and measure the related risks;
- Examine all possibilities, effectiveness, reliability, and expenditure to attain the best results for the company concerned

Knowledge required by the OHS professional in the US include:

- Constitutional and case law controlling safety, health, and the environment
- Operational procedures to plan/develop safe work practices
- Safety, health and environmental sciences
- Design of hazard control systems (i.e. fall protection, scaffoldings)
- Design of recordkeeping systems that take collection into account, as well as storage, interpretation, and dissemination
- Mathematics and statistics
- Processes and systems for attaining safety through design

Some skills required by the OHS professional in the US include (but are not limited to):

- Understanding and relating to systems, policies and rules
- Holding checks and having control methods for possible hazardous exposures
- Mathematical and statistical analysis
- Examining manufacturing hazards
- Planning safe work practices for systems, facilities, and equipment

- Understanding and using safety, health, and environmental science information for the improvement of procedures
- Interpersonal communication skills

Differences between Countries and Regions

Because different countries take different approaches to ensuring occupational safety and health, areas of OSH need and focus also vary between countries and regions. Similar to the findings of the ENHSPO survey conducted in Australia, the Institute of Occupational Medicine in the UK found that there is a need to put greater emphasis on work-related illness in the UK. In contrast, in Australia and the US, a major responsibility of the OHS professional is to keep company directors and managers aware of the issues that they face in regards to occupational health and safety principles and legislation. However, in some other areas of Europe, it is precisely this which has been lacking: "Nearly half of senior managers and company directors do not have an up-to-date understanding of their health and safety-related duties and responsibilities."

Identifying Safety and Health Hazards

Hazards, Risks, Outcomes

The terminology used in OSH varies between countries, but generally speaking:

- A hazard is something that can cause harm if not controlled.
- The outcome is the harm that results from an uncontrolled hazard.
- A risk is a combination of the probability that a particular outcome will occur and the severity of the harm involved.

"Hazard", "risk", and "outcome" are used in other fields to describe e.g. environmental damage, or damage to equipment. However, in the context of OSH, "harm" generally describes the direct or indirect degradation, temporary or permanent, of the physical, mental, or social well-being of workers. For example, repetitively carrying out manual handling of heavy objects is a hazard. The outcome could be a musculoskeletal disorder (MSD) or an acute back or joint injury. The risk can be expressed numerically (e.g. a 0.5 or 50/50 chance of the outcome occurring during a year), in relative terms (e.g. "high/medium/low"), or with a multi-dimensional classification scheme (e.g. situation-specific risks).

Hazard Identification

Hazard identification or assessment is an important step in the overall risk assessment and risk management process. It is where individual work hazards are identified, assessed and controlled/eliminated as close to source (location of the hazard) as reasonably as possible. As technology, resources, social expectation or regulatory requirements change, hazard analysis focuses controls more closely toward the source of the hazard. Thus hazard control is a dynamic program of prevention. Hazard-based programs also have the advantage of not assigning or implying there are "acceptable risks" in the workplace. A hazard-based program may not be able to eliminate all risks, but neither does it accept "satisfactory" – but still risky – outcomes. And as those who calculate and manage the risk are usually managers while those exposed to the risks are a different group, workers, a hazard-based approach can by-pass conflict inherent in a risk-based approach.

The information that needs to be gathered from sources should apply to the specific type of work from which the hazards can come from. As mentioned previously, examples of these sources include interviews with people who have worked in the field of the hazard, history and analysis of past incidents, and official reports of work and the hazards encountered. Of these, the personnel interviews may be the most critical in identifying undocumented practices, events, releases, hazards and other relevant information. Once the information is gathered from a collection of sources, it is recommended for these to be digitally archived (to allow for quick searching) and to have a physical set of the same information in order for it to be more accessible. One innovative way to display the complex historical hazard information is with a historical hazards identification map, which distills the hazard information into an easy to use graphical format.

Risk Assessment

Modern occupational safety and health legislation usually demands that a risk assessment be carried out prior to making an intervention. It should be kept in mind that risk management requires risk to be managed to a level which is as low as is reasonably practical.

This assessment should:

- Identify the hazards
- Identify all affected by the hazard and how
- Evaluate the risk
- Identify and prioritize appropriate control measures

The calculation of risk is based on the likelihood or probability of the harm being realized and the severity of the consequences. This can be expressed mathematically as a quantitative assessment (by assigning low, medium and high likelihood and severity with integers and multiplying them to obtain a risk factor), or qualitatively as a description of the circumstances by which the harm could arise.

The assessment should be recorded and reviewed periodically and whenever there is a significant change to work practices. The assessment should include practical recommendations to control the risk. Once recommended controls are implemented, the risk should be re-calculated to determine if it has been lowered to an acceptable level. Generally speaking, newly introduced controls should lower risk by one level, i.e., from high to medium or from medium to low.

Contemporary Developments

On an international scale, the World Health Organization (WHO) and the International Labour Organization (ILO) have begun focusing on labour environments in developing nations with projects such as Healthy Cities. Many of these developing countries are stuck in a situation in which their relative lack of resources to invest in OSH leads to increased costs due to work-related illnesses and accidents. As a 2007 Factsheet from the European Agency for Safety and Health at Work states: "Countries with less developed OSH systems spend a far higher percentage of GDP on work-related injury and illness – taking resources away from more productive activities ... The ILO estimates that work-related illness and accidents cost up to 10% of GDP in Latin America, compared with just 2.6% to 3.8% in the EU." There is continued use of asbestos, a notorious hazard, in some developing countries. So asbestos-related disease is, sadly, expected to continue to be a significant problem well into the future.

Nanotechnology

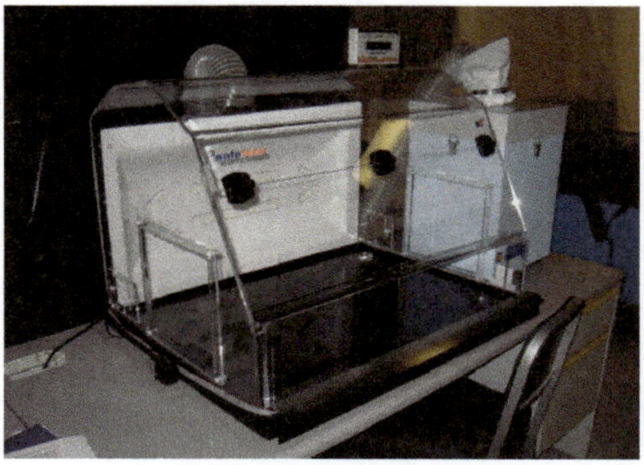

A nanomaterial containment hood, an example of an engineering control used to protect workers handling them on a regular basis.

Nanotechnology is an example of a new, relatively unstudied technology. A Swiss survey of one hundred thirty eight companies using or producing nanoparticulate matter in 2006 resulted in forty completed questionnaires. Sixty five per cent of respondent companies stated they did not have a formal risk assessment process for dealing with nanoparticulate matter. Nanotechnology already presents new issues for OSH professionals that will only become more difficult as nanostructures become more complex. The size of the particles renders most containment and personal protective equipment ineffective. The toxicology values for macro sized industrial substances are rendered inaccurate due to the unique nature of nanoparticulate matter. As nanoparticulate matter decreases in size its relative surface area increases dramatically, increasing any catalytic effect or chemical reactivity substantially versus the known value for the macro substance. This presents a new set of challenges in the near future to rethink contemporary measures to safeguard the health and welfare of employees against a nanoparticulate substance that most conventional controls have not been designed to manage.

Occupational Health Disparities

Occupational health disparities refer to differences in occupational injuries and illnesses that are closely linked with demographic, social, cultural, economic, and/or political factors.

Education

There are multiple levels of training applicable to the field of occupational safety and health (OSH). Programs range from individual non-credit certificates, focusing on specific areas of concern, to full doctoral programs. The University of Southern California was one of the first schools in the US to offer a Ph.D. program focusing on the field. Further, multiple master's degree programs exist, such as that of the Indiana State University who offer a master of science (MS) and a master of arts (MA) in OSH. Graduate programs are designed to train educators, as well as, high-level practitioners. Many OSH generalists focus on undergraduate studies; programs within schools, such as that of the University of North Carolina's online Bachelor of Science in Environmental Health and Safety, fill a large majority of hygienist needs. However, smaller companies often don't have full-time safety specialists on staff, thus, they appoint a current employee to the responsibility. Individuals finding themselves in positions such as these, or for those enhancing marketability in the job-search and promotion arena, may seek out a credit certificate program. For example, the University of Connecticut's online OSH Certificate, provides students familiarity with overarching concepts through a 15-credit (5-course) program. Programs such as these are often adequate tools in building a strong educational platform for new safety managers with a minimal outlay of time and money. Further, most hygienists seek certification by organizations which train in specific areas of concentration, focusing on isolated workplace hazards. The American Society for Safety Engineers (ASSE), American Board of Industrial Hygiene (ABIH), and American Industrial Hygiene Association (AIHA) offer individual certificates on many different subjects from forklift operation to waste disposal and are the chief facilitators of continuing education in the OSH sector. In the U.S. the training of safety professionals is supported by National Institute for Occupational Safety and Health through their NIOSH Education and Research Centers. In Australia, training in OSH is available at the vocational education and training level, and at university undergraduate and postgraduate level. Such university courses may be accredited by an Accreditation Board of the Safety Institute of Australia. The Institute has produced a Body of Knowledge which it considers is required by a generalist safety and health professional, and offers a professional qualification based on a four-step assessment.

World Day for Safety and Health at Work

On April 28 The International Labour Organisation celebrates "World Day for Safety and Health" to raise awareness of safety in the workplace. Occurring annually since 2003, each year it focuses on a specific area and bases a campaign around the theme.

Occupational Health Psychology

Occupational health psychology (OHP) is an interdisciplinary area of psychology that is concerned with the health and safety of workers. OHP addresses a number of major topic areas including the impact of occupational stressors on physical and mental health, the impact of involuntary unemployment on physical and mental health, work-family balance, workplace violence and other forms of mistreatment, accidents and safety, and interventions designed to improve/protect worker health. OHP emerged from two distinct disciplines within applied psychology, namely, health psychology and industrial and organizational psychology, as well as occupational medicine. OHP has also been informed by other disciplines including industrial sociology, industrial engineering, and economics, as well as preventive medicine and public health. OHP is concerned with the relationship of psychosocial workplace factors to the development, maintenance, and promotion of workers' health and that of their families. Thus the field's focus is work-related factors that can lead to injury, disease, and distress.

Historical Overview

Origins

The Industrial Revolution prompted thinkers, such as Karl Marx with his theory of alienation, to concern themselves with the nature of work and its impact on workers. Taylor's (1911) *Principles of Scientific Management* as well as Mayo's research in the late 1920s and early 1930s on workers at the Hawthorne Western Electric plant helped to inject the impact of work on workers into the subject matter psychology addresses. The creation in 1948 of the Institute for Social Research (ISR) at the University of Michigan was important because of its research on occupational stress and employee health.

Research in the U.K. by Trist and Bamforth (1951) suggested the reduction in autonomy that accompanied organizational changes in English coal mining operations adversely affected worker morale. Arthur Kornhauser's work in the early 1960s on the mental health of automobile workers in Michigan also contributed to the development of the field. A 1971 study by Gardell examined the impact of work organization on mental health in Swedish pulp and paper mill workers and engineers. Research on the impact of unemployment on mental health was conducted at the University of Sheffield's Institute of Work Psychology. In 1970 Kasl and Cobb documented the impact of unemployment on blood pressure in U.S. factory workers.

Recognition as a Field of Study

The term "occupational health psychology" first appeared in print in 1986 when Everly advocated for psychologists' role in workplace health promotion. In 1988, in response to a dramatic increase in the number of stress-related worker compensation claims in the U.S., the National Institute for Occupational Safety and Health (NIOSH) added psychological factors to its list of factors "leading occupational health risk". When this change was coupled with an increased recognition of the impact of stress on a range of problems in the workplace, NIOSH found that their stress-related programs were significantly increasing in prominence. In 1990, Raymond et al. argued that the time has come for doctoral-level psychologists to get interdisciplinary OHP training, integrating health psychology with public health, because creating healthy workplaces should be a goal for the field.

Emergence as a Discipline

Established in 1987, *Work & Stress* is the first and "longest established journal in the fast developing discipline that is occupational health psychology". Three years later, the American Psychological Association (APA) and NIOSH jointly organized the first international Work, Stress, and Health conference in Washington, DC. The conference has since become a biannual OHP meeting. In 1996, the *Journal of Occupational Health Psychology* was published by APA. That same year, the International Commission on Occupational Health created the Work Organisation and Psychosocial Factors (ICOH-WOPS) scientific committee, which focused primarily on OHP. In 1999, the European Academy of Occupational Health Psychology (EA-OHP) was established at the first European Workshop on Occupational Health Psychology in Lund, Sweden. That workshop is considered to be the first EA-OHP conference, the first of a continuing series of conferences EA-OHP organizes and devotes to OHP research and practice.

In 2000 the informal International Coordinating Group for Occupational Health Psychology (ICGOHP) was founded for the purpose of facilitating OHP-related research, education, and practice as well as coordinating international conference scheduling. Also in 2000, *Work & Stress* became associated with the EA-OHP. In 2005, the Society for Occupational Health Psychology (SOHP) was established in the United States. In 2008, SOHP joined with APA and NIOSH in co-sponsoring the Work, Stress, and Health conferences. In 2017, SOHP began to publish an OHP-related journal *Occupational Health Science*.

Research Methods

The main purpose of OHP research is to understand how working conditions affect worker health, use that knowledge to design interventions to protect and improve worker health, and evaluate the effectiveness of such interventions. The research methods used in OHP are similar to those used in other branches of psychology.

Standard Research Designs

Self-report survey methodology is the most used approach in OHP research. Cross-sectional designs are commonly used; case-control designs have been employed much less frequently. Longitudinal designs including prospective cohort studies and experience sampling studies can examine relationships over time. OHP-related research devoted to evaluating health-promoting workplace interventions has relied on quasi-experimental designs and, less commonly, experimental approaches.

Quantitative Methods

Statistical methods commonly used in other areas of psychology are also used in OHP-related research. Statistical methods used include structural equation modeling and hierarchical linear modeling (HLM; also known as multilevel modeling). HLM can better adjust for similarities between employees and is especially well suited to evaluating the lagged impact of work stressors on health outcomes; in this research context HLM can help minimize censoring and is well-suited to experience sampling studies. Meta-analyses have been used to aggregate data (modern approaches to meta-analyses rely on HLM), and draw conclusions across multiple studies.

Qualitative Research Methods

Qualitative research methods include interviews, focus groups, and self-reported, written descriptions of stressful incidents at work. First-hand observation of workers on the job has also been used, as has participant observation.

Research Topics

Important Theoretical Models in OHP Research

Three influential theoretical models in OHP research are the demand-control-support, demand-resources, and effort-reward imbalance models.

Demand-control-support Model

The most influential model in OHP research has been the original demand-control model. According to the model, the combination of low levels of work-related decision latitude (i.e., autonomy and control over the job) combined with high workloads (high levels of work demands) can be particularly harmful to workers (they can lead to "job strain," a term representing the combination of low decision latitude and high workload leading to poorer mental or physical health). The model suggests not only that these two job factors are related to poorer health but that high levels of decision latitude on the job will buffer or reduce the adverse health impact of high levels of demands. Research has clearly supported the idea that decision latitude and demands relate to strains, but research findings about buffering have been mixed with only some studies providing support. The demand-control model asserts that job control can come in two broad forms: 'skill discretion' and 'decision authority'. Skill discretion refers to the level of skill and creativity required on the job and the flexibility an employee is permitted in deciding what skills to use (e.g. opportunity to use skills, similar to job variety). Decision authority refers to employees being able to make decisions about their work (e.g., having autonomy). These two forms of job control are traditionally assessed together in a composite measure of decision latitude; there is, however, some evidence that the two types of job control may not be similarly related to health outcomes.

About a decade after Karasek first introduced the demand-control model, Johnson, Hall, and Theorell (1989), in the context of research on heart disease, extended the model to include social isolation. Johnson et al. labeled the combination of high levels of demands, low levels of control, and low levels of coworker support "iso-strain." The resulting expanded model has been labeled the demand–control–support (DCS) model. Research that followed the development of this model has suggested that one or more of the components of the DCS model (high psychological workload, low control, and lack of social support), if not the exact combination represented by iso-strain, have adverse effects of physical and mental health.

Job Demands-resources Model

An alternative model, the job demands-resources (JD-R) model, grew out of the DCS model. In the JD-R model, the category of demands (workload) remains more or less the same as in the DCS model although the JD-R model more specifically includes physical demands. Resources, however, are defined as job-relevant features that help workers achieve work-related goals, lessen job demands, or stimulate personal growth. Control and support as per the DCS model are subsumed under resources. Resources can be external (provided by the organization) or internal (part of a worker's personal make-up). In addition to control and support, resources encompassed by the model can also include physical equipment, software, performance feedback from supervisors, the worker's own coping strategies, etc. There has not, however, been as much research on the JD-R model as there has been on the constituents of the DC or DCS model.

Effort-reward Imbalance Model

After the DCS model, the, perhaps, second most influential model in OHP research has been the effort-reward imbalance (ERI) model. It links job demands to the rewards employees receive for the job. That model holds that high work-related effort coupled with low control over job-related intrinsic (e.g., recognition) and extrinsic (e.g., pay) rewards triggers high levels of activation in neurohormonal pathways that, cumulatively, are thought to exert adverse effects on mental and physical health.

Occupational Stress and Cardiovascular Disease

A number of work-related, psychosocial factors have been linked to cardiovascular disease (CVD).

Cardiovascular Disease

Research has identified health-behavioral and biological factors that are related to increased risk for CVD. These risk factors include smoking, obesity, low density lipoprotein (the "bad" cholesterol), lack of exercise, and blood pressure. Psychosocial working conditions are also risk factors for CVD. In a case-control study involving two large U.S. data sets, Murphy (1991) found that hazardous work situations, jobs that required vigilance and responsibility for others, and work that required attention to devices were related to increased risk for cardiovascular disability. These included jobs in transportation (e.g., air traffic controllers, airline pilots, bus drivers, locomotive engineers, truck drivers), preschool teachers, and craftsmen. Among 30 studies involving men and women, most have found an association between workplace stressors and CVD.

Fredikson, Sundin, and Frankenhaeuser (1985) found that reactions to psychological stressors include increased activity in the brain axes which play an important role in the regulation of blood pressure, particularly ambulatory blood pressure. A meta-analysis and systematic review involving 29 samples linked job strain to elevated ambulatory blood pressure. Belkić et al. (2000) found that many of the 30 studies covered in their review revealed that decision latitude and psychological workload exerted independent effects on CVD; two studies found synergistic effects, consistent with the strictest version of the demand-control model. A review of 17 longitudinal studies having reasonably high internal validity found that 8 showed a significant relation between the combination of low latitude and high workload (the job strain condition) and CVD and 3 more showed a nonsignificant relation. The findings, however, were clearer for men than for women, on whom data were more sparse. In a massive ($n > 197{,}000$) longitudinal study that combined data from 13 independent studies, Kivimäki et al. (2012) found that, controlling for other risk factors, the combination of high levels of demands and low control at baseline increased the risk of CVD in initially healthy workers by between 20 and 30% over a follow-up period that averaged 7.5 years. In this study the effects were similar for men and women.

There is evidence that, consistent with the ERI model, high work-related effort coupled with low control over job-related rewards adversely affects cardiovascular health. At least five studies of men have linked effort-reward imbalance with CVD.

Job Loss and Cardiovascular Health

Research has suggested that job loss adversely affects cardiovascular health as well as health in general.

Job-related Burnout and Cardiovascular Health

There is evidence from a prospective study that job-related burnout, controlling for traditional risk factors, such as smoking and hypertension, increases the risk of coronary heart disease over the course of the next three and a half years in workers who were initially disease-free.

Musculoskeletal Disorders

Musculoskeletal disorders (MSDs) involve injury and pain to the joints and muscles of the body. Approximately 2.5 million workers in the US suffer from MSDs, which is the third most common cause of disability and early retirement for American workers. In Europe MSDs are the most often reported workplace health problem. The development of musculoskelelatal problems cannot be solely explained in the basis of biomechanical factors (e.g., repetitive motion) although such factors are important contributors. There has been evidence that psychosocial workplace factors (e.g., job strain) also contribute to the development of musculoskeletal problems.

Workplace Mistreatment

There are many forms of workplace mistreatment ranging from relatively minor incivility to serious cases of bullying and violence.

Workplace Incivility

Workplace incivility has been defined as "low-intensity deviant behavior with ambiguous intent to harm the target....Uncivil behaviors are characteristically rude and discourteous, displaying a lack of regard for others". Incivility is distinct from violence. Examples of workplace incivility include insulting comments, denigration of the target's work, spreading false rumors, social isolation, etc. A summary of research conducted in Europe suggests that workplace incivility is common there. In research on more than 1000 U.S. civil service workers, more than 70% of the sample experienced workplace incivility in the past five years. Compared to men, women were more exposed to incivility; incivility was associated with psychological distress and reduced job satisfaction.

Abusive Supervision

Abusive supervision is the extent to which a supervisor engages in a pattern of behavior that harms subordinates.

Workplace Bullying

Although definitions of workplace bullying vary, it involves a repeated pattern of harmful behaviors directed towards an individual by one or more others who have more power than the target. Workplace bullying is sometimes termed *mobbing*.

Sexual Harassment

Sexual harassment is behavior that denigrates or mistreats an individual due to his or her gender, creates an offensive workplace, and interferes with an individual being able to do the job.

Workplace Violence

Workplace violence is a significant health hazard for employees.

-Nonfatal assault-

Most workplace assaults are nonfatal, with an annual physical assault rate of 6% in the U.S. Assaultive behavior in the workplace often produces injury, psychological distress, and economic loss. One study of California workers found a rate of 72.9 non-fatal, officially documented assaults per 100,000 workers per year, with workers in the education, retail, and health care sectors subject to excess risk. A Minnesota workers' compensation study found that women workers had a twofold higher risk of being injured in an assault than men, and health and social service workers, transit workers, and members of the education sector were at high risk for injury compared to workers in other economic sectors. A West Virginia workers' compensation study found that workers in the health care sector and, to a lesser extent, the education sector were at elevated risk for assault-related injury. Another workers' compensation study found that excessively high rates of assault-related injury in schools, healthcare, and, to a lesser extent, banking. In addition to the physical injury that results from being a victim of workplace violence, individuals who witness such violence without being directly victimized are at increased risk for experiencing adverse effects, as found in a study of Los Angeles teachers.

-Homicide-

In 1996 there were 927 work-associated homicides in the United States, in a labor force that numbered approximately 132,616,000. The rate works out to be about 7 homicides per million workers for the one year. Men are more likely to be victims of workplace homicide than women.

Mental Disorder

Research has found that psychosocial workplace factors are among the risk factors for a number of categories of mental disorder.

Alcohol Abuse

Workplace factors can contribute to alcohol abuse and dependence of employees. Rates of abuse can vary by occupation, with high rates in the construction and transportation industries as well as among waiters and waitresses. Within the transportation sector, heavy truck drivers and material movers were at especially high risk. A prospective study of ECA subjects who were followed one year after the initial interviews provided data on newly incident cases of alcohol abuse and dependence. The study found that workers in jobs that combined low control with high physical demands were at increased risk of developing alcohol problems although the findings were confined to men.

Depression

Using data from the ECA study, Eaton, Anthony, Mandel, and Garrison (1990) concluded that members of three occupational groups, lawyers, secretaries, and special education teachers (but not other types of teachers) showed elevated rates of *DSM-III* major depression, adjusting for social demographic factors. The ECA study involved representative samples of American adults from five U.S. geographical areas, providing relatively unbiased estimates of the risk of mental disorder by occupation; however, because the data were cross-sectional, no conclusions bearing on cause-and-effect relations are warranted. Evidence from a Canadian prospective study indicated that individuals in the highest quartile of occupational stress (high-strain jobs as per the demand-control model) are at increased risk of experiencing an episode of major depression. A meta-analysis that pooled the results of 11 well-designed longitudinal studies indicated that a number of facets of the psychosocial work environment (e.g., low decision latitude, high psychological workload, lack of social support at work, effort-reward imbalance, and job insecurity) increase the risk of common mental disorders such as depression.

Personality Disorders

Depending on the diagnosis, severity and individual, and the job itself, personality disorders can be associated with difficulty coping with work or the workplace, potentially leading to problems with others by interfering with interpersonal relationships. Indirect effects also play a role; for example, impaired educational progress or complications outside of work, such as substance abuse and co-morbid mental disorders, can plague sufferers. However, personality disorders can also bring about above-average work abilities by increasing competitive drive or causing the sufferer to exploit his or her co-workers.

Schizophrenia

In a case-control study, Link, Dohrenwend, and Skodol found that, compared to depressed and well control subjects, schizophrenic patients were more likely to have had jobs, prior to their first episode of the disorder, that exposed them to "noisesome" work characteristics (e.g., noise, humidity, heat, cold, etc.). The jobs tended to be of higher status than other blue collar jobs, suggesting that downward drift in already-affected individuals does not account for the finding. One explanation involving a diathesis-stress model suggests that the job-related stressors helped precipitate the first episode in already-vulnerable individuals. There is some supporting evidence from the Epidemiologic Catchment Area (ECA) study.

Psychological Distress

Longitudinal studies have suggested adverse working conditions can contribute to the development of psychological distress. Psychological distress refers to negative affect, without the individuals necessarily meeting criteria for a psychiatric disorder. Psychological distress is often expressed in affective (depressive), psychophysical or psychosomatic (e.g., headaches, stomach aches, etc.), and anxiety symptoms. The relation of adverse working conditions to psychological distress is thus an important avenue of research. Job satisfaction is also related to negative health outcomes.

Psychosocial Working Conditions

Parkes (1982) studied the relation of working conditions to psychological distress in British student nurses. She found that in this "natural experiment," student nurses experienced higher levels of distress and lower levels of job satisfaction in medical wards than in surgical wards; compared to surgical wards, medical wards make greater affective demands on the nurses. In another study, Frese (1985) concluded that objective working conditions give rise to subjective stress and psychosomatic symptoms in blue collar German workers. In addition to the above studies, a number of other well-controlled longitudinal studies have implicated work stressors in the development of psychological distress and reduced job satisfaction.

Unemployment

A comprehensive meta-analysis involving 86 studies indicated that involuntary job loss is linked to increased psychological distress. The impact of involuntary unemployment was comparatively weaker in countries that had greater income equality and better social safety nets. The research evidence also indicates that poorer mental health slightly, but significantly, increases the risk of later job loss.

Economic Insecurity

Some OHP research is concerned with (a) understanding the impact of economic crises on individuals' physical and mental health and well-being and (b) calling attention to personal and organizational means for ameliorating the impact of the crisis. Economic insecurity contributes, at least partly, to psychological distress and work-family conflict. Ongoing job insecurity, even in the absence of job loss, is related to higher levels of depressive symptoms, psychological distress, and worse overall health.

Work-family

Employees must balance their working lives with their home lives. Work–family conflict is a situation in which the demands of work conflict with the demands of family, making it difficult to adequately do both, giving rise to distress.

Workplace Interventions

A number of stress management interventions have emerged that have shown demonstrable effects in reducing job stress. Cognitive behavioral interventions have tended to have greatest impact on stress reduction.

Industrial Organizations

OHP interventions often concern both the health of the individual and the health of the organization. Adkins (1999) described the development of one such intervention, an organizational health center (OHC) at a California industrial complex. The OHC helped to improve both organizational and individual health as well as help workers manage job stress. Innovations included labor-management partnerships, suicide risk reduction, conflict mediation, and occupational mental health support. OHC practitioners also coordinated their services with previously underutilized local community services in the same city, thus reducing redundancy in service delivery.

Hugentobler, Israel, and Schurman (1992) detailed a different, multi-layered intervention in a mid-sized Michigan manufacturing plant. The hub of the intervention was the Stress and Wellness Committee (SWC) which solicited ideas from workers on ways to improve both their well-being and productivity. Innovations the SWC developed included improvements that ensured two-way communication between workers and management and reduction in stress resulting from diminished conflict over issues of quantity versus quality. Both the interventions described by Adkins and Hugentobler et al. had a positive impact on productivity.

OHP Research at the National Institute for Occupational Safety and Health

Currently there are efforts under way at NIOSH to help reduce the incidence of preventable disorders (e.g., sleep apnea) among heavy-truck and tractor-trailer drivers and, concomitantly, the life-threatening accidents to which the disorders lead, improve the health and safety of workers who are assigned to shift work or who work long hours, and reduce the incidence of falls among iron workers.

Military and First Responders

The Mental Health Advisory Teams of the United States Army employ OHP-related interventions with combat troops. OHP also has a role to play in interventions aimed at helping first responders.

Modestly Scaled Interventions

Schmitt (2007) described three different modestly scaled OHP-related interventions that helped workers abstain from smoking, exercise more frequently, and shed weight. Other OHP interventions include a campaign to improve the rates of hand washing, an effort to get workers to walk more often, and a drive to get employees to be more compliant with regard to taking prescribed medicines. The interventions tended reduce organization health-care costs.

Health Promotion

Organizations can play a role in the health behavior of employees by providing resources to encourage healthy behavior in areas of exercise, nutrition, and smoking cessation.

Prevention

Although the dimensions of the problem of workplace violence vary by economic sector, one sector, education, has had some limited success in introducing programmatic, psychologically-based efforts to reduce the level of violence. Research suggests that there continue to be difficulties in successfully "screening out applicants [for jobs] who may be prone to engaging in aggressive behavior," suggesting that aggression-prevention training of existing employees may be an alternative to screening. Only a small number of studies evaluating the effectiveness of training programs to reduce workplace violence currently exist.

Accidents and Safety

Psychological factors are an important factor in occupational accidents that can lead to injury and death of employees. An important influence on the incidence of accidents is the organization's safety climate that is employees' shared beliefs about how supervisors reward and support safety behavior.

Prevention Through Design

Prevention through design (PtD), also called safety by design usually in Europe, is the concept of applying methods to minimize occupational hazards early in the design process, with an emphasis on optimizing employee health and safety throughout the life cycle of materials and processes. It is a concept and movement that encourages construction or product designers to "design out" health and safety risks during design development. The concept supports the view that along with quality, programme and cost; safety is determined during the design stage. It increases the cost-effectiveness of enhancements to occupational safety and health.

This method for reducing workplace safety risks lessens workers' reliance on personal protective equipment, which is the least effective of the hierarchy of hazard control.

Background

Each year in the U.S., 55,000 people die from work-related injuries and diseases, 294,000 are made sick, and 3.8 million are injured. The annual direct and indirect costs have been estimated to range from $128 billion to $155 billion. Recent studies in Australia indicate that design is a significant contributor in 37% of work-related fatalities; therefore, the successful implementation of prevention through design concepts can have substantial impacts on worker health and safety. The National Institute for Occupational Safety and Health in the United States considers PtD to be "the most effective and reliable type" of prevention of occupational injuries.

Within Europe, construction designers are legally bound to design out risks during design development to reduce hazards in the construction and end use phases via the Mobile Worksite Directive (also known as CDM regulations in the UK). The concept supports this legal requirement. Some Notified Bodies provide testing and design verification services to ensure compliance with the safety standards defined in regulation codes such as the American Society of Mechanical Engineers. Many non-governmental organizations have been established to support this aim, principally in the UK, Australia and the United States.

History

While engineering as a rule factors human safety into the design process, a modern appraisal of specific links to design and workers' safety can be seen in efforts beginning in the 1800s. Trends included the widespread implementation of guards for machinery, controls for elevators, and boiler safety practices. This was followed by enhanced design for ventilation, enclosures, system monitors, lockout/tagout controls, and hearing protectors. More recently, there has been the development of chemical process safety, ergonomically engineered tools, chairs, and work stations, lifting devices, retractable needles, latex-free gloves, and a parade of other safety devices and processes. The National Institute for Occupational Health and Safety has started an initiative called "Buy Quiet", which uses elements of Prevention through Design to encourage companies to buy quieter machienery, thereby reducing occupational hearing loss for their workers.

Integration

Prevention through design represents a shift in approach for on-the-job safety. It involves evaluating potential risks associated with processes, structures, equipment, and tools. It takes into consideration the construction, maintenance, decommissioning, and disposal or recycling of waste material.

The idea of redesigning job tasks and work environments has begun to gain momentum in business and government as a cost-effective means to enhance occupational safety and health. Many U.S. companies openly support PtD concepts and have developed management practices to implement them. Other countries are actively promoting PtD concepts as well. The United Kingdom began requiring construction companies, project owners, and architects to address safety and health during the design phase of projects in 1994. Australia developed the Australian National OHS Strategy 2002–2012, which set "eliminating hazards at the design stage" as one of five national priorities. As a result, the Australian Safety and Compensation Council (ASCC) developed the Safe Design National Strategy and Action Plans for Australia encompassing a wide range of design areas.

Personal Protective Equipment

Personal protective equipment (PPE) refers to protective clothing, helmets, goggles, or other garments or equipment designed to protect the wearer's body from injury or infection. The hazards addressed by protective equipment include physical, electrical, heat, chemicals, biohazards, and airborne particulate matter. Protective equipment may be worn for job-related occupational safety and health purposes, as well as for sports and other recreational activities. "Protective clothing" is applied to traditional categories of clothing, and "protective gear" applies to items such as pads, guards, shields, or masks, and others.

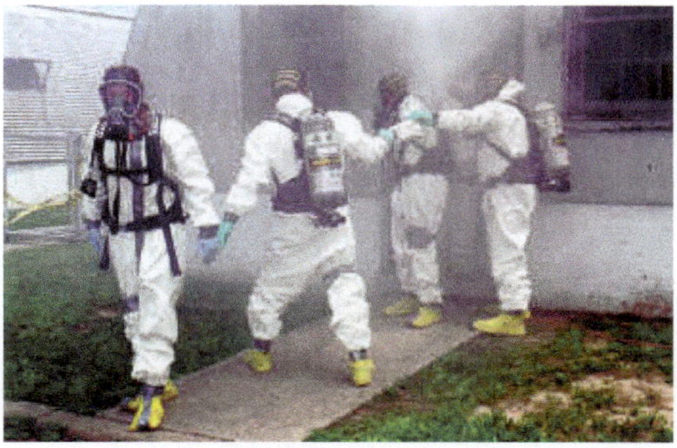

Drug Enforcement Administration (DEA) agents wearing Level B hazmat suits

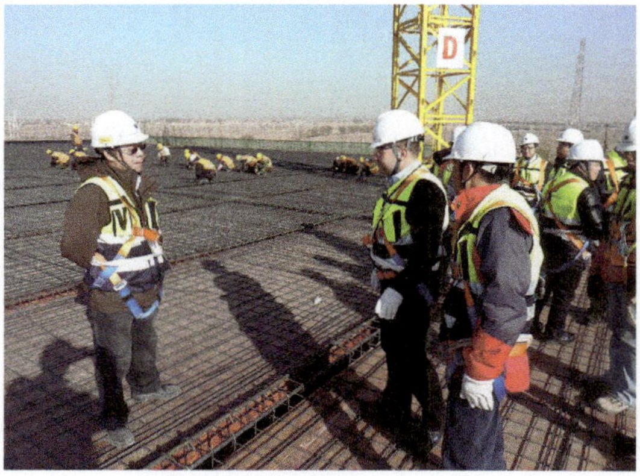

Safety equipment and supervisor instructions at a construction site

The purpose of personal protective equipment is to reduce employee exposure to hazards when engineering controls and administrative controls are not feasible or effective to reduce these risks to acceptable levels. PPE is needed when there are hazards present. PPE has the serious limitation that it does not eliminate the hazard at source and may result in employees being exposed to the hazard if the equipment fails.

Any item of PPE imposes a barrier between the wearer/user and the working environment. This can create additional strains on the wearer; impair their ability to carry out their work and create significant levels of discomfort. Any of these can discourage wearers from using PPE correctly, therefore placing them at risk of injury, ill-health or, under extreme circumstances, death. Good ergonomic design can help to minimise these barriers and can therefore help to ensure safe and healthy working conditions through the correct use of PPE.

Practices of occupational safety and health can use hazard controls and interventions to mitigate workplace hazards, which pose a threat to the safety and quality of life of workers. The hierarchy of hazard controls provides a policy framework which ranks the types of hazard controls in terms of absolute risk reduction. At the top of the hierarchy are elimination and substitution, which remove the hazard entirely or replace the hazard with a safer alternative. If elimination or substitution measures cannot apply, engineering controls and administrative controls, which seek to design safer mechanisms and coach safer human behavior, are implemented. Personal protective equipment ranks last on the hierarchy of controls, as the workers are regularly exposed to the hazard, with a barrier of protection. The hierarchy of controls is important in acknowledging that, while personal protective equipment has tremendous utility, it is not the desired mechanism of control in terms of worker safety.

Types

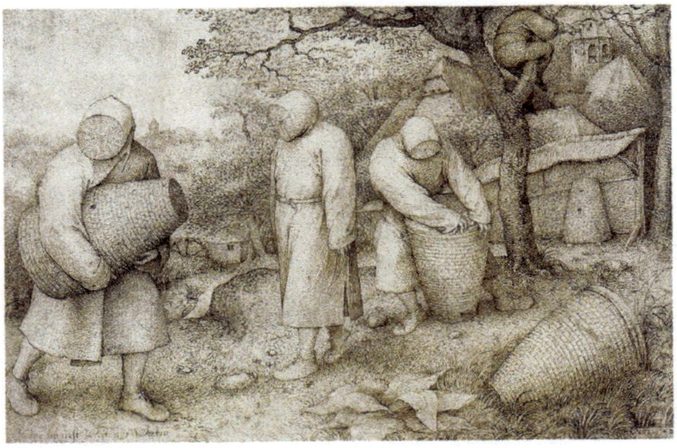

A 1568 painting depicting beekeepers in protective clothing

Personal protective equipment can be categorized by the area of the body protected, by the types of hazard, and by the type of garment or accessory. A single item, for example boots, may provide multiple forms of protection: a steel toe cap and steel insoles for protection of the feet from crushing or puncture injuries, impervious rubber and lining for protection from water and chemicals, high reflectivity and heat resistance for protection from radiant heat, and high electrical resistivity for protection from electric shock. The protective attributes of each piece of equipment must be compared with the hazards expected to be found in the workplace. More breathable types of personal protective equipment may not lead to more contamination but do result in greater user satisfaction.

Respirators

Respirators serve to protect the user from breathing in contaminants in the air, thus preserving the health of one's respiratory tract. There are two main types of respirators. One type functions by filtering out chemicals and gases, or airborne particles, from the air breathed by the user. The filtration may be either passive or active (powered). Gas masks and particulate respirators are examples of this type of respirator. A second type protects users by providing clean, respirable air from another source. This type includes airline respirators and self-contained breathing apparatus (SCBA). In work environments, respirators are relied upon when adequate ventilation is not available or other engineering control systems are not feasible or inadequate.

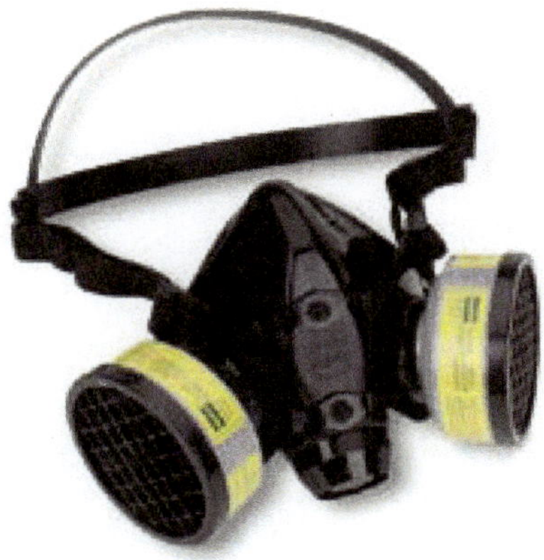

Air-purifying respirator

In the United Kingdom, an organization that has extensive expertise in respiratory protective equipment is the Institute of Occupational Medicine. This expertise has been built on a long-standing and varied research programme that has included the setting of workplace protection factors to the assessment of efficacy of masks available through high street retail outlets.

The Health and Safety Executive (HSE), NHS Health Scotland and Healthy Working Lives (HWL) have jointly developed the RPE (Respiratory Protective Equipment) Selector Tool, which is web-based. This interactive tool provides descriptions of different types of respirators and breathing apparatuses, as well as "dos and don'ts" for each type.

In the United States, The National Institute for Occupational Safety and Health (NIOSH) provides recommendations on respirator use, in accordance to NIOSH federal respiratory regulations 42 CFR Part 84. The National Personal Protective Technology Laboratory (NPPTL) of NIOSH is tasked towards actively conducting studies on respirators and providing recommendations.

Skin Protection

Occupational skin diseases such as contact dermatitis, skin cancers, and other skin injuries and infections are the second-most common type of occupational disease and can be very costly. Skin hazards, which lead to occupational skin disease, can be classified into four groups. Chemical agents can come into contact with the skin through direct contact with contaminated surfaces, deposition of aerosols, immersion or splashes. Physical agents such as extreme temperatures and ultraviolet or solar radiation can be damaging to the skin over prolonged exposure. Mechanical trauma occurs in the form of friction, pressure, abrasions, lacerations and contusions. Biological agents such as parasites, microorganisms, plants and animals can have varied effects when exposed to the skin.

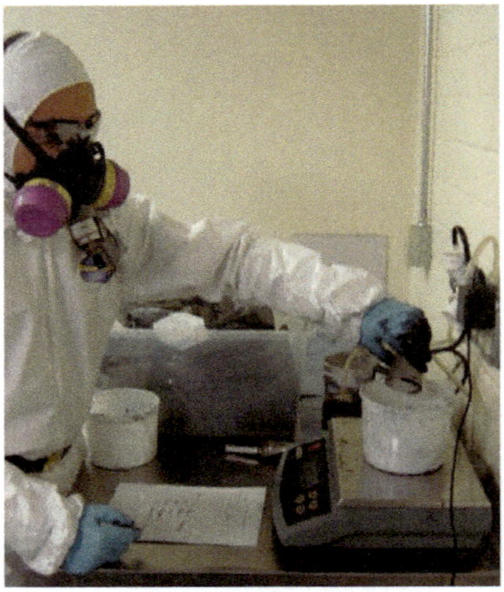

A worker wearing a respirator, lab coat, and gloves while weighing carbon nanotubes

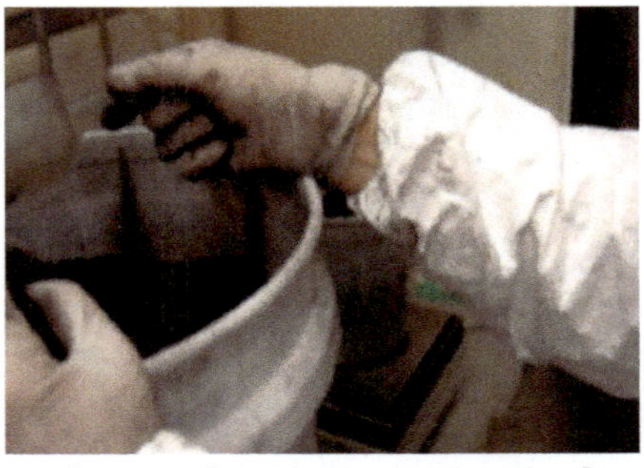

This is an incorrect use of personal protective equipment, because the gap between the glove and the lab coat exposes the wrist to hazardous materials.

Any form of PPE that acts as a barrier between the skin and the agent of exposure can be considered skin protection. Because much work is done with the hands, gloves are an essential item in providing skin protection. Some examples of gloves commonly used as PPE include rubber gloves, cut-resistant gloves, chainsaw gloves and heat-resistant gloves. For sports and other recreational activities, many different gloves are used for protection, generally against mechanical trauma.

Other than gloves, any other article of clothing or protection worn for a purpose serve to protect the skin. Lab coats for example, are worn to protect against potential splashes of chemicals. Face shields serve to protect one's face from potential impact hazards, chemical splashes or possible infectious fluid.

Eye Protection

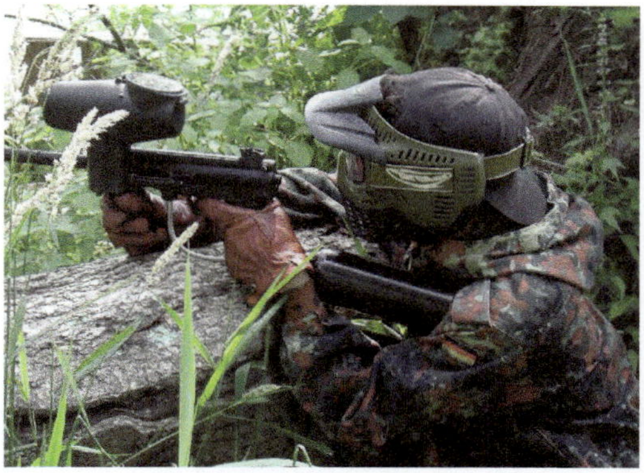

A paintball player wearing appropriate eye protection against impact.

Each day, about 2000 US workers have a job-related eye injury that requires medical attention. Eye injuries can happen through a variety of means. Most eye injuries occur when solid particles such as metal slivers, wood chips, sand or cement chips get into the eye. Smaller particles in smokes and larger particles such as broken glass also account for particulate matter-causing eye injuries. Blunt force trauma can occur to the eye when excessive force comes into contact with the eye. Chemical burns, biological agents, and thermal agents, from sources such as welding torches and UV light, also contribute to occupational eye injury.

While the required eye protection varies by occupation, the safety provided can be generalized. Safety glasses provide protection from external debris, and should provide side protection via a wrap-around design or side shields.

- Goggles provide better protection than safety glasses, and are effective in preventing eye injury from chemical splashes, impact, dusty environments and welding. Goggles with high air flow should be used to prevent fogging.
- Face shields provide additional protection and are worn over the standard eyewear; they also provide protection from impact, chemical, and blood-borne hazards.

- Full-facepiece respirators are considered the best form of eye protection when respiratory protection is needed as well, but may be less effective against potential impact hazards to the eye.
- Eye protection for welding is shaded to different degrees, depending on the specific operation.

Hearing Protection

Industrial noise is often overlooked as an occupational hazard, as it is not visible to the eye. Overall, about 22 million workers in the United States are exposed to potentially damaging noise levels each year. Occupational hearing loss accounted for 14% of all occupational illnesses in 2007, with about 23,000 cases significant enough to cause permanent hearing impairment. About 82% of occupational hearing loss cases occurred to workers in the manufacturing sector. The Occupational Safety and Health Administration establishes occupational noise exposure standards. NIOSH recommends that worker exposures to noise be reduced to a level equivalent to 85 dBA for eight hours to reduce occupational noise-induced hearing loss.

PPE for hearing protection consists of earplugs and earmuffs. Workers who are regularly exposed to noise levels above the NIOSH recommendation should be furnished hearing protection by the employers, as they are a low-cost intervention.

Protective Clothing and Ensembles

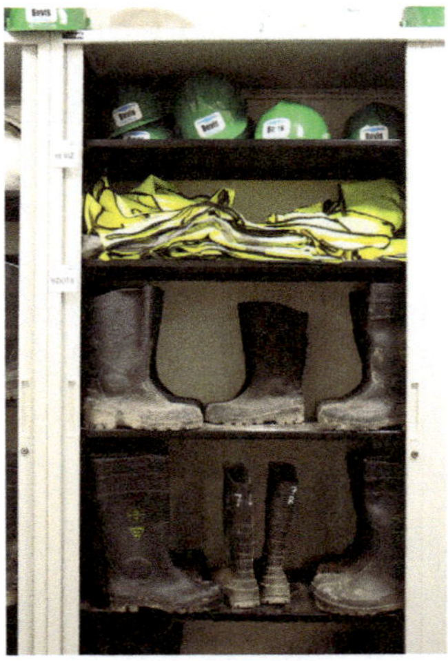

Locker containing personal protective equipment

This form of PPE is all-encompassing and refers to the various suits and uniforms worn to protect the user from harm. Lab coats worn by scientists and ballistic vests worn by law enforcement officials, which are worn on a regular basis, would fall into this category. Entire sets of PPE, worn together in a combined suit, are also in this category.

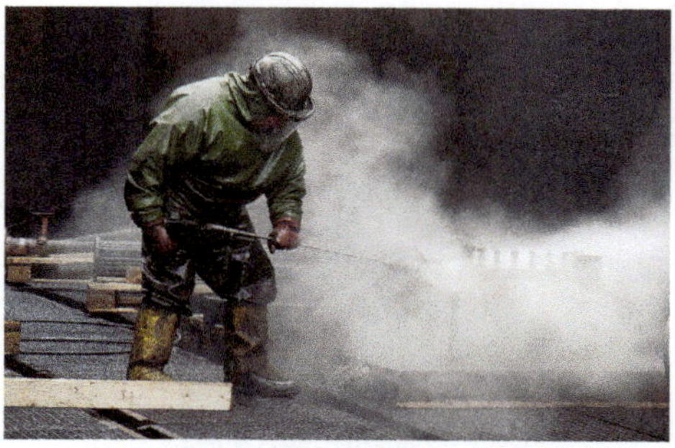

A complete PPE ensemble worn during high pressure cleaning work

Ensembles

Below are some examples of ensembles of personal protective equipment, worn together for a specific occupation or task, to provide maximum protection for the user.

- Chainsaw protection (especially a helmet with face guard, hearing protection, kevlar chaps, anti-vibration gloves, and chainsaw safety boots).
- Bee-keepers wear various levels of protection depending on the temperament of their bees and the reaction of the bees to nectar availability. At minimum most bee keepers wear a brimmed hat and a veil made of fine mesh netting. The next level of protection involves leather gloves with long gauntlets and some way of keeping bees from crawling up one's trouser legs. In extreme cases, specially fabricated shirts and trousers can serve as barriers to the bees' stingers.
- Diving equipment, for underwater diving, constitutes equipment such as a diving helmet or diving mask, an underwater breathing apparatus, and a diving suit.
- Firefighters wear PPE designed to provide protection against fires and various fumes and gases. PPE worn by firefighters include bunker gear, self-contained breathing apparatus, a helmet, safety boots, and a PASS device.

In Sports

Participants in sports often wear protective equipment. Studies performed on the injuries of professional athletes, such as that on NFL players, question the effectiveness of existing personal protective equipment.

Limits of the Definition

The definition of what constitutes as personal protective equipment varies by country. In the United States, the laws regarding PPE also vary by state. In 2011, workplace safety complaints were brought against Hustler and other adult film production companies by the AIDS Healthcare Foundation, leading to several citations brought by Cal/OSHA. The failure to use condoms by adult film stars was a violation of Cal/OSHA's Blood borne Pathogens Program, Personal Protective Equipment. This example shows that personal protective equipment can cover a variety of occupations in the United States, and has a wide-ranging definition.

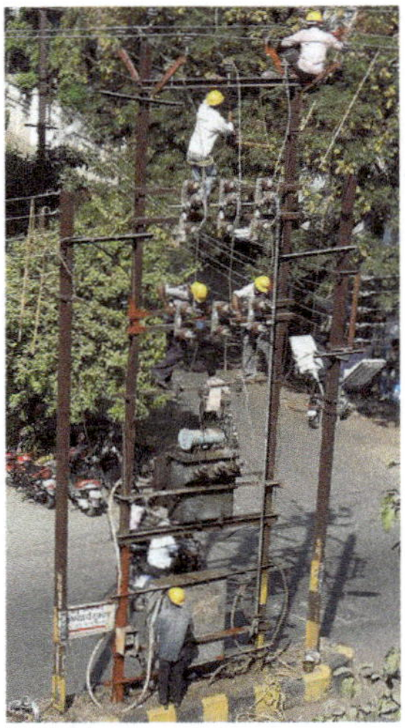

Workers using personal protective equipment while painting poles. While basic head protection is present, no engineering fall protection systems appear to be in place.

Legislation in the European Union

At the European Union level, personal protective equipment is governed by Directive 89/686/EEC on personal protective equipment (PPE). The Directive is designed to ensure that PPE meets common quality and safety standards by setting out basic safety requirements for personal protective equipment, as well as conditions for its placement on the market and free movement within the EU single market. It covers 'any device or appliance designed to be worn or held by an individual for protection against one or more health and safety hazards'. The directive was adopted on 21 January 1989 and came into force on 1 July 1992. The European Commission additionally allowed for a transition period until 30 June 1995 to give companies sufficient time to adapt to the legislation. After this date, all PPE placed on the market in EU Member States was required to comply with the requirements of Directive 89/686/EEC and carry the CE Marking.

Article 1 of Directive 89/686/EEC defines personal protective equipment as any device or appliance designed to be worn or held by an individual for protection against one or more health and safety hazards. PPE which falls under the scope of the Directive is divided into three categories:

- Category I: simple design (e.g. gardening gloves, footwear, ski goggles)
- Category II: PPE not falling into category I or III (e.g. personal flotation devices, dry and wet suits)
- Category III: complex design (e.g. respiratory equipment, harnesses)

Directive 89/686/EEC on personal protective equipment does not distinguish between PPE for professional use and PPE for leisure purposes.

Personal protective equipment falling within the scope of the Directive must comply with the basic health and safety requirements set out in Annex II of the Directive. To facilitate conformity with these requirements, harmonized standards are developed at the European or international level by the European Committee for Standardization (CEN, CENELEC) and the International Organization for Standardization in relation to the design and manufacture of the product. Usage of the harmonized standards is voluntary and provides presumption of conformity. However, manufacturers may choose an alternative method of complying with the requirements of the Directive.

Personal protective equipment excluded from the scope of the Directive includes:

- PPE designed for and used by the armed forces or in the maintenance of law and order;
- PPE for self-defence (e.g. aerosol canisters, personal deterrent weapons);
- PPE designed and manufactured for personal use against adverse atmospheric conditions (e.g. seasonal clothing, umbrellas), damp and water (e.g. dish-washing gloves) and heat;
- PPE used on vessels and aircraft but not worn at all times;
- helmets and visors intended for users of two- or three-wheeled motor vehicles.

The European Commission is currently working to revise Directive 89/686/EEC. The revision will look at the scope of the Directive, the conformity assessment procedures and technical requirements regarding market surveillance. It will also align the Directive with the New Legalislative Framework. The European Commission is likely to publish its proposal in 2013. It will then be discussed by the European Parliament and Council of the European Union under the ordinary legislative procedure before being published in the Official Journal of the European Union and becoming law.

Construction Site Safety

Construction work is a hazardous land-based job. Some construction site jobs include: building houses, roads, tree forts, workplaces and repair and maintain infrastructures. This work includes many hazardous task and conditions such as working with height, excavation, noise, dust, power tools and equipment. The most common fatalities are caused by the fatal four: falls, struck by object, electrocutions and caught-in/between. Construction work has been increasing in developing and undeveloped countries over the past few years. With an increase in this type of work occupational fatalities have increased. Occupational fatalities are individuals that pass way while on the job or performing work related tasks. Within the field of construction it is important to have safe construction sites.

Construction Fatality Rates

In 2014, the United States had 4,679 fatal occupational injuries; incidence rate of 3.3 per 100,000 full-time employed workers. In the same year, fatal work injuries in construction and extraction occupations increased 5%. One in five workers died in 2014 were due to construction related deaths. Construction has about 6% of U.S. workers, but 17% of the fatalities - the largest number of fatalities reported for any industry sector. In the United Kingdom, the construction industry is responsible for 31% of fatalities at work and 10% of major workplace injuries. I In South Africa there are 150 fatalities and approximately 400 injuries each year related to construction sites. In Brazil, the incidence rate for all occupational fatalities is 3.6 per 100,000. (Little to no information regarding construction fatalities could be found in Asia, South American, Africa, and Antarctic). The chart below contains more countries and the rate of construction site fatalities.

Chart of Fatality Rates in Different Countries

Country/Region	Fatalities (per Annum per 100,000 Workers)	Year
Australia	1.85	2013
Canada	8.7	2008
Europe	23.0	2012
France	2.64	2012
Finland	5.9	2008
Germany	5.0	2008
Ireland	9.80	2013
India	10.0	2008
Norway	3.3	2008
Sweden	5.8	2008
Switzerland	4.2	2008
United Kingdom	1.62	2015
United States of America	9.8	2014
Israel	12.12	2015

Nature of Hazards

Hazards to Construction Workers

The leading safety hazards on construction sites include: falls, caught between objects, electrocutions, and struck by objects. All four of those hazards have caused injuries and deaths throughout the world of construction sites. Failures in hazard identification are often due to limited or improper training and supervision of the construction site workers. Examples of areas were there are limited training includes: tasks in design for safety, safety inspection, and monitoring safety. Failure in any of these areas can result in an increased risk in exposing workers to harm in the construction environment.

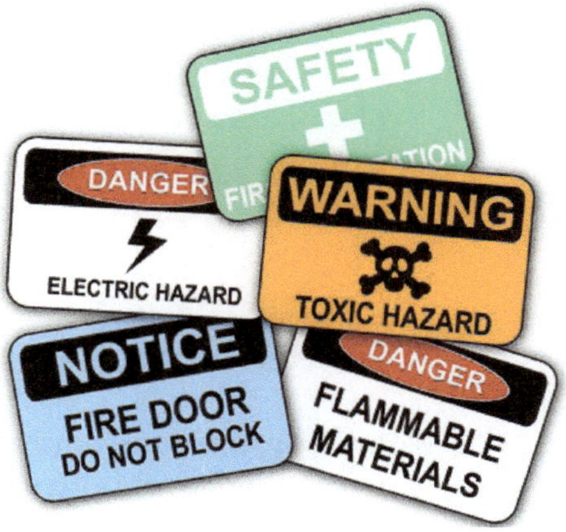

Various workplace safety signs commonly used at construction sites and industrial work environments.

Falls are the leading cause of injury in the construction industry, is particularly for elder and untrained construction workers. In the Occupational Safety and Health Administration (OSHA) Handbook (29 CFR) used by the United States, fall protection is needed in areas including but are not limited to: ramps, runways, and other walkways; excavations; hoist areas; holes; form-work; leading edge work; unprotected sides and edges; overhand bricklaying and related work; roofing; precast erection; wall openings; residential construction; and other walking/working surfaces. Other countries have regulations and guidelines for fall protections to prevent injuries and deaths. Therefore, it is important that construction sites are safe as possible for the workers.

Motor vehicle crashes are another major safety hazard on construction sites. It is important to be cautious while operation motor vehicles or equipment on the site. Motor vehicles should have a service brake system, emergency brake system, and a parking brake system. All vehicles must be equipped with an audible warning system if the operator chooses to use it. Vehicles must have windows and doors, power windshield wipers, and have a clear view of site from the rear window. All employees should be properly trained before using motor vehicles and the equipment.

Employees on construction sites also need to be aware of dangers on the ground. The hazards of cables running across roadways were often seen, until cable ramp equipment was invented to protect hoses and other equipment which had to be laid out. Other hazards found on construction site includes: asbestos, solvents, noise, and manual handling activities.

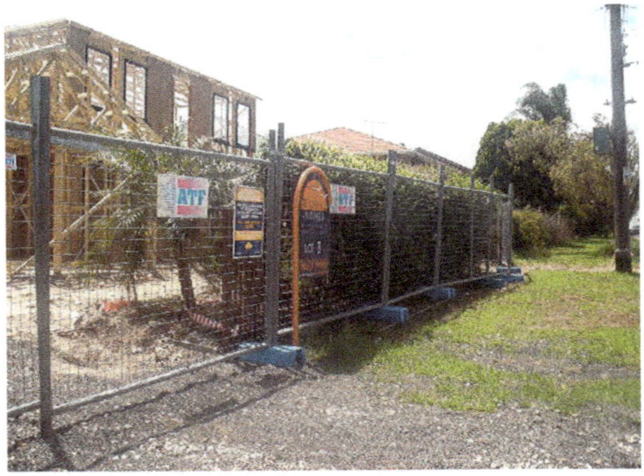

Temporary fencing on a building site in Sydney, Australia.

Education and Safety

Construction workers need to be properly trained and educated on the task or job before working, which will assist in preventing injuries and deaths. There are many methods on training construction workers. One method is coaching construction site foremen to include safety in their daily verbal exchanges with workers to reduce work-related accidents. It is important that the workers use the same speaking language to assure for the best communication. In recent years, apart from traditional face to face safety knowledge sharing, the popularity of mobile apps make knowledge sharing through apps possible

Another method is that all workers know how to properly work and use electronics, conveyors, skid-steer, trucks, aerial lifts, and other equipment on the construction site. Also, equipment on the job site must be properly maintain and inspected regularly before and after each shift. The equipment inspection system will help the operator to make sure that the machine is mechanically sound and in safe operating conditions. An employee should be assigned to inspect equipment to insure proper safety is being met. Equipment should have lights and reflectors if intended for night use. The glass in the cab of the equipment must be safety glass in some countries. The equipment must be used for their intended task at all times on the job site to insure safety of the workers.

Each construction site should have a construction site manager. A construction site manager's is an occupational health and safety specialist who designs and implements safety regulations to minimize injuries and accidents on construction sites. He or she also is in charge of conducting daily safety audits and inspections to ensure compliance with government regulations. Most construction site managers have an entry level experience or higher degree.

Before any excavation takes place, the contractor is responsible to notify all applicable companies that excavation work is being performed. During excavation, the contractor is responsible for providing a safe work environment for employees and pedestrians. Access and Egress is also an important part of excavation safety. Ramps used by equipment must be designed by a person, qualified in structural design. No person is allowed to cross underneath or stand underneath any loading or digging equipment. Employees are to remain at a safe distance from all equipment while it is operational. Employees that have training and education in the above areas will benefit their co-workers and themselves on the construction site.

Road Construction Safety

The American Recovery and Reinvestment Act of 2009 created over 12,600 road construction projects, over 10,000 of which are currently in progress. Workers in highway work zones are exposed to a variety of hazards and face risk of injury and death from construction equipment as well as passing motor vehicles. Workers on foot are exposed to passing traffic, often at high speeds, while workers who operate construction vehicles are at risk of injury due to overturn, collision, or being caught in running equipment. Regardless of the task assigned, construction workers work in conditions in poor lighting, poor visibility, inclement weather, congested work areas, high volume traffic and speeds. In 2011, there were a total of 119 fatal occupation fatalities in road construction sites. In 2010 there were 37,476 injuries in work zones, about 20,000 of those injuries are construction workers. Causes of road work site injuries include being struck by objects, trucks or mobile equipment (35%), falls or slips (20%), overexertion (15%), transportation incidents (12%), and exposure to harmful substances or environments (5%). Causes of fatalities include getting hit by trucks (58%), mobile machinery (22%), and automobiles (13%).

Media Safety Campaigns Road construction safety remains a priority among workers. Several states have implemented campaigns addressing construction zone dangers and encouraging motorists to use caution when driving through work zones. National Work Zone Safety Awareness Week is held yearly. The national event began in 1999 and has gained popularity and media attention each year since. The purpose of the event is to draw national attention to motorist and worker safety issues in work zones.

Preventing Accidents and Improving Safety

Site preparation will aid in preventing injury and death on construction sites. Site preparation includes removing all the debris existing on the site, leveling the ground, filling holes, cutting off tree roots, and marking gas, water, and electric pipelines. This process improves the safety on the construction site. Another prevention methods on the construction site is to provide scaffold that is rigid and sufficient to carry its own weight plus four times the maximum intended load without settling or displacement.

Ways to Prevent Injuries and Improve safety Include:

1. Management safety
2. Integrate safety as a part of the job
3. Create accountability at all levels
4. Take safety into account during the project planning process
5. Make sure the contractors are pre-qualified for safety
6. Make sure the workers are properly trained in appropriate areas
7. Have a fall protection system
8. Prevent and address substance abuse to employees
9. Make safety a part of everyday conversation
10. Review accidents and near misses, as well as regular inspections
11. Innovative safety training, e.g. adoption of virtual reality in training
12. Replace some of the works by robots (many workers may worry that this will decrease their employment rate).
13. Adoption of BIM with three dimensional printing to make the building model first before put into real practice

The employees or employers are responsible for providing fall protection systems and to ensure the use of systems. Fall protection can be provided by guardrail systems, safety net systems, personal fall arrest systems, positioning device systems, and warning line systems. Making sure that ladders are long enough to safely reach the work area to prevent injury. Stairway, treads, and walkways must be free of dangerous objects, debris and materials. A registered professional engineer should design a protective system for trenches 20 feet deep or greater for safety reasons. To prevent injury with a crane, they should be inspected for any damage. Plus the operator should know the maximum weight of the load that the crane is to lift. All operators should be trained and certified to ensure that they operate forklifts safely.

Operational Excellence Model to improve safety for construction organizations

There are 13 safety drivers associated with this model to improve safety for construction organizations:

1. Recognition & Reward
2. Employee Engagement

3. Subcontractor Management
4. Training & Competence
5. Risk Awareness, Management & Tolerance
6. Learning Organization
7. Human Performance
8. Transformational Leadership
9. Shared Values, Beliefs, and Assumptions
10. Strategic Safety Communication
11. Just & Fair Practices and Procedures
12. Worksite Organization
13. Owner's Role

Each safety driver mentioned above has some sub-elements attributed to it.

Personal Protective Equipment

Hard hats and steel-toe boots are perhaps the most common personal protective equipment worn by construction workers around the world. A risk assessment may deem that other protective equipment is appropriate, such as gloves, goggles, or high-visibility clothing.

Hazards to Non-workers

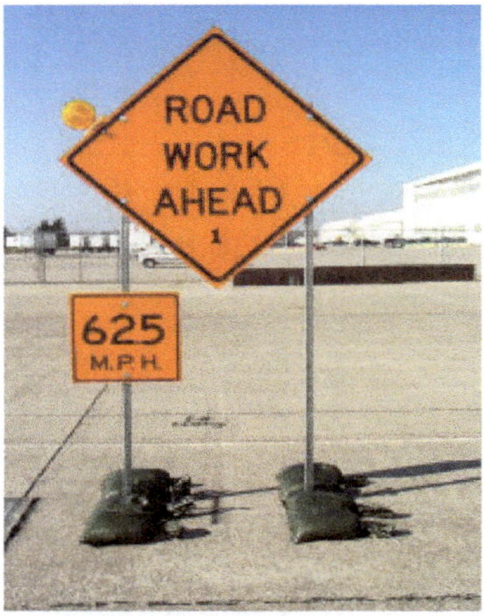

This sign and advisory plate penetrated the wind-shield and roof of a car in a side-impact test crash. A safer sign would have stiffer uprights, no advisory plate and the flashing light would be moved to the point of the sign to spread the impact force.

Many construction sites cannot completely exclude non-workers. Road construction sites must often allow traffic to pass through. This places non-workers at some degree of risk.

Road construction sites are blocked-off and traffic is redirected. The sites and vehicles are protected by signs and barricades. However, sometimes even these signs and barricades can be a hazard to vehicle traffic. For example, improperly designed barricades can cause cars that strike them to roll over or even be thrown into the air. Even a simple safety sign can penetrate the wind-shield or roof of a car if hit from certain angles. The majority of death in construction are caused by hazards relating to construction activity. However, many deaths are also caused by non construction activities, such as electrical hazards. A notable example of this occurred when Andy Roberts, a father of four, was killed while changing a light bulb at a construction site when he came into contact with a loose bare wire that was carrying two thousand volts of electricity and died. (August 1988 New York (U.S.A)). Events like this motivated the passing of further safety laws relating to non construction activities such as electrical work laws.

Applicable Laws

Under European Union Law, there are European Union Directives in place to protect workers, notably Directive 89/391 (the Framework Directive) and Directive 92/57 (the Temporary and Mobile Sites Directive). This legislation is transposed into the Member States and places requirements on employers (and others) to assess and protect workers health and safety.

In the United States, the Occupational Safety and Health Administration (OSHA) sets and enforces standards concerning workplace safety and health. In the United States, efforts have been made in the first decade of the 21st century to improve safety for both road workers and drivers in construction zone. In 2004, Title 23 Part 630 Subpart J of the Code of Federal Regulations was updated by congress to include new regulations that direct state agencies to systematically create and adopt comprehensive plans to address safety in road construction zones that receive federal funding.

In the United Kingdom, the Health and Safety Executive (HSE) is responsible for standards enforcement, while in Northern Ireland, the Health and Safety Executive for Northern Ireland (HSENI) is responsible. In Ireland, the Health and Safety Authority (HSA) is responsible for standards and enforcement.

In Europe, the European Agency for Safety and Health at Work coordinates actions at the EU and national levels and the Directorate-General for Employment, Social Affairs and Inclusion is responsible for regulation at the EU level.

In the United States, the Department of Labor Occupational Safety and Health Administration (OSHA), implemented the Final Rule to Improve Tracking of Workplace Injuries and Illnesses. The new rule, has went into effect January 1, 2017. It requires employers to submit incident data electronically to OSHA. This data will enable OSHA to use enforcement and compliance assistance resources more efficiently. The amount of data required varies by company and industry.

Agricultural Safety and Health

Agricultural safety and health is an aspect of occupational safety and health in the agricultural workplace. It specifically addresses the health and safety of farmers, farm workers, and their families.

Risk

The agriculture industry is one of the most dangerous occupations and has led to thousands of deaths due to work-related injuries in the US. In 2011 the fatality rate for farmworkers was 7 times higher than that of all the workers in the private industry, a difference of 24.9 deaths for every 100,000 people as opposed to 3.5 deaths for every 100,000 people in the private industry. The National Institute for Occupational Safety and Health (NIOSH) estimated that 374 farmers and farmworkers died due to a work-related injury in 2012, tractor overturns being the number one cause death. An average of 113 youth between the ages of 16-19 years die annually from agriculture related injuries (1995-2002). About 167 farmworkers each day are affected by a lost-work-time injury in which 5% of them suffer from permanent damage. Non-fatal injuries that farmworkers are at high risk for include work-related lung problems, hearing loss due to noise, skin diseases, various cancers due to exposure to certain chemicals as well as prolonged exposure to the sun.

Laws and Regulation

Unlike other industries that impose labor laws and occupational safety and health regulations in the workplace, agriculture deals with diverse production, large labor force and an array of environmental conditions that makes it difficult to address. The Occupational Safety and Health Administration (OSHA) has approved 28 state plans that are required to include standards and enforcement programs. These standards and programs can have requirements that are different or more strict than OSHA's but they must be in the very least as effective as OSHA's.

Occupational Medicine

Occupational medicine, especially until 1960 called industrial medicine, is the branch of medicine which deals with the maintenance of health in the workplace, including the prevention and treatment of diseases and injuries, and also promotes productivity and social adjustment.

It is thus the branch of clinical medicine most active in the field of occupational health and safety. OM specialists work to ensure that the highest standards of occupational health and safety can be achieved and maintained. While OM may involve a wide number of disciplines, it centers on preventive medicine and the management of illness, injury, and disability related to the workplace. Occupational physicians must have a wide knowledge of clinical medicine and be competent in a number of important areas. They often advise international bodies, governmental and state agencies, organizations and trade unions. There are contextual links to physical medicine and rehabilitation and to insurance medicine.

Mission

Occupational medicine aims to prevent diseases and promote wellness among workers. Occupational health physicians must:

- Have knowledge of potential hazards in the workplace including toxic properties of materials used.
- Be able to evaluate employee fitness for work.
- Be able to diagnose and treat occupational disease and injury.
- Know about rehabilitation methods, health education, and government laws and regulations concerning workplace health.
- Be able to manage health service delivery.

OM can be described as:

"work that combines clinical medicine, research, and advocacy for people who need the assistance of health professionals to obtain some measure of justice and health care for illnesses they suffer as a result of companies pursuing the biggest profits they can make, no matter what the effect on workers or the communities they operate in."

Mine Safety

Safety has long been a concern in the mining business, especially in underground mining. The Courrières mine disaster, Europe's worst mining accident, involved the death of 1,099 miners in Northern France on March 10, 1906. This disaster was surpassed only by the Benxihu Colliery accident in China on April 26, 1942, which killed 1,549 miners. While mining today is substantially safer than it was in previous decades, mining accidents still occur. Government figures from China indicate that 5,000 Chinese miners die in accidents each year, while other reports have suggested a figure as high as 20,000. Mining accidents continue worldwide, including accidents causing dozens of fatalities at a time such as the 2007 Ulyanovskaya Mine disaster in Russia, the 2009 Heilongjiang mine explosion in China, and the 2010 Upper Big Branch Mine disaster in the United States.

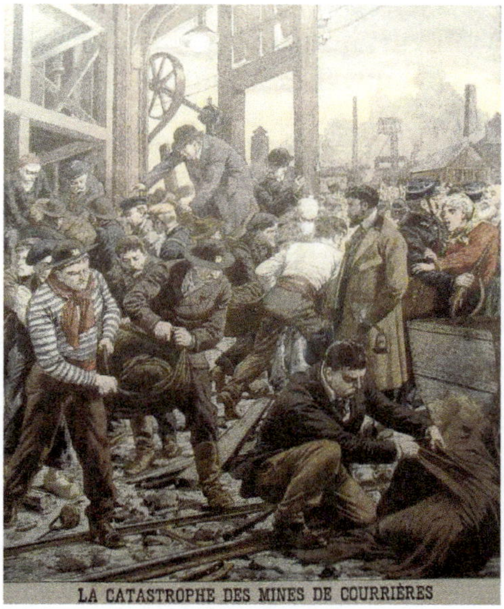

Le Petit Journal illustration of the Courrières mine disaster

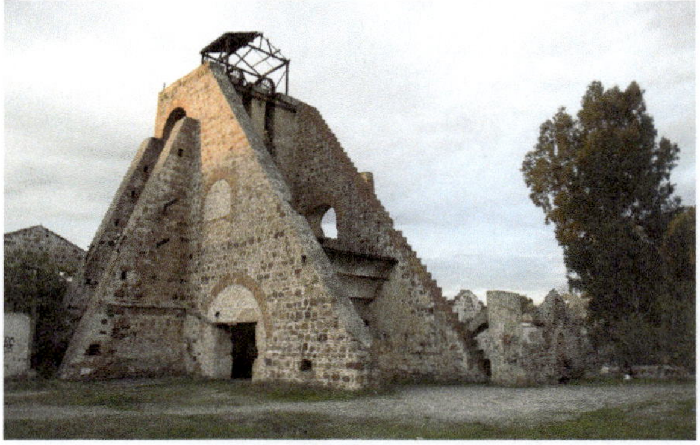

Remnants of pit "San Vicente" in Linares, Jaén, Spain. On its last day of operation, in 1967, six workers died in an elevator accident.

Hazards and Prevention

Ventilation

Mining ventilation is a significant safety concern for many miners. Poor ventilation inside sub-surface mines causes exposure to harmful gases, heat, and dust, which can cause illness, injury, and death. The concentration of methane and other airborne contaminants underground can generally be controlled by dilution (ventilation), capture before entering the host air stream (methane drainage), or isolation (seals and stoppings). A ventilation system is set up to force a stream of air through the working areas of the mine. The air circulation necessary for effective ventilation of a mine is generated by one or more large mine fans, usually located above ground. Air flows in one direction only, making circuits through the mine such that each main work area constantly receives a supply of fresh air. Watering down in coal mines also helps to keep dust levels down: by spraying the machine with water and filtering the dust-laden water with a scrubber fan, miners can successfully trap the dust.

Gases in mines can poison the workers or displace the oxygen in the mine, causing asphyxiation. For this reason, the U.S. Mine Safety and Health Administration requires that groups of miners in the United States carry gas detection equipment that can detect common gases, such as CO, O_2, H_2S, CH_4, as well as calculate % Lower Explosive Limit. Regulation requires that all production stop if there is a concentration of 1.4% of flammable gas present. Additionally, further regulation is being requested for more gas detection as newer technology such as nanotechnology is introduced.

Gas Ignition

Ignited methane gas is a common source of explosions in coal mines, which in turn can initiate more extensive coal dust explosions. For this reason, rock dusts such as limestone dust are spread throughout coal mines to diminish the chances of coal dust explosions as well as to limit the extent of potential explosions, in a process known as rock dusting. Coal dust explosions can also begin independently of methane gas explosions. Frictional heat and sparks generated by mining equipment can ignite both methane gas and coal dust. For this reason, water is often used to cool rock-cutting sites.

Noise

Miners utilize equipment strong enough to break through extremely hard layers of the Earth's crust. This equipment, combined with the closed work space in which underground miners work, can cause hearing loss. For example, a roof bolter (commonly used by mine roof bolter operators) can reach sound power levels of up to 115 dB. Combined with the reverberant effects of underground mines, a miner without proper hearing protection is at a high risk for hearing loss. By age 50, nearly 90% of U.S. coal miners have some hearing loss, compared to only 10% among workers not exposed to loud noises. Roof bolters are among the loudest machines, but auger miners, bulldozers, continuous mining machines, front end loaders, and shuttle cars and trucks are also among those machines most responsible for excessive noise in mine work.

The preferred prevention strategy involves engineering controls to eliminate noise sources. Administrative controls and hearing protection can also be used when engineering controls are not feasible.

Cave-ins and Rock Falls

Since mining entails removing dirt and rock from its natural location, thereby creating large empty pits, rooms, and tunnels, cave-ins as well as ground and rock falls are a major concern within mines. Modern techniques for timbering and bracing walls and ceilings within sub-surface mines have reduced the number of fatalities due to cave-ins, but ground falls continue to represent up to 50% of mining fatalities. Even in cases where mine collapses are not instantly fatal, they can trap mine workers deep underground. Cases such as these often lead to high-profile rescue efforts, such as when 33 Chilean miners were trapped deep underground for 69 days in 2010.

Heat Exposure

High temperatures and humidity may result in heat-related illnesses, including heat stroke, which can be fatal. The presence of heavy equipment in confined spaces also poses a risk to miners. To improve the safety of mine workers, modern mines use automation and remote operation including, for example, such equipment as automated loaders and remotely operated rockbreakers. However, despite modern improvements to safety practices, mining remains a dangerous occupation throughout the world.

Use of Explosives

Explosives are used in mines for constructive purposes, but can be hazardous if proper safety measures are not taken. For example, flyrock can be ejected beyond the blast site, causing personal injuries and damage to property.

Dust Exposure

In coal mining, the extraction, crushing, and transport of coal can generate significant amounts of airborne respirable (extremely fine) coal dust. Dust less than 10 microns in size (cannot be seen with the eye). In non-coal mining, stone, and sand and gravel mining operations and for particular occupations in coal mines, the respirable silica dust created during mining is the primary concern. Respirable dust can cause long-term lung problems. Respirable coal dust can cause coal workers' pneumoconiosis (also known as miners lung or black lung disease), respirable silica dust can cause silicosis, lung cancer, and chronic obstructive pulmonary disease. Elongate mineral particles can lead to asbestosis, lung cancer, and mesothelioma.

Abandoned Mines

There are upwards of 560,000 abandoned mines on public and privately owned lands in the United States alone. Abandoned mines may be dangerous to anyone who attempts to explore them without proper knowledge and safety training.

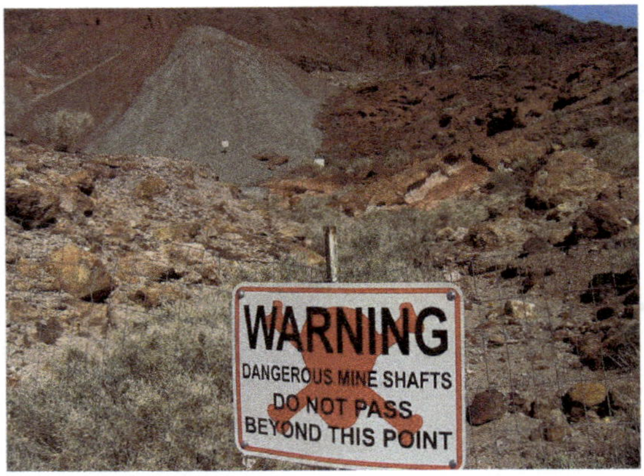
WARNING
DANGEROUS MINE SHAFTS
DO NOT PASS
BEYOND THIS POINT

Warning sign near a dangerous area filled with open mineshafts, Calico Ghost Town, California.

Regulations

In the United States, the Mine Safety and Health Administration (MSHA) develops and enforces regulations to ensure mining safety. Additionally, the National Institute for Occupational Safety and Health (NIOSH) researches occupational health issues related to mining.

Occupational Hygiene

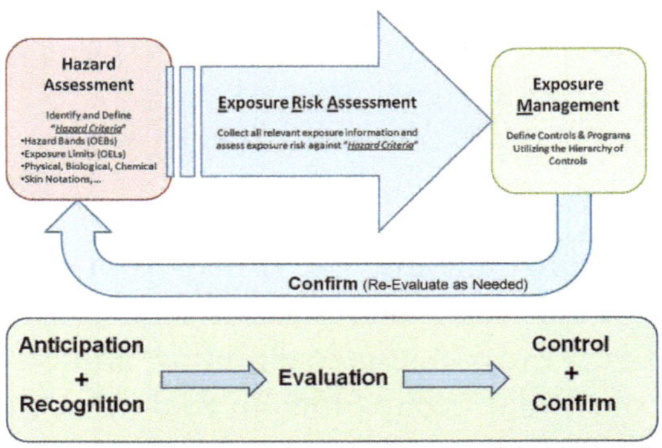

Fundamental Elements of Industrial Hygiene (ERAM Model)

Illustration of Exposure Risk Assessment and Management related to anticipation, recognition, evaluation, control and confirm.

Occupational hygiene (United States: industrial hygiene (IH)) is the anticipation, recognition, evaluation, control and prevention of hazards from work that may result in injury, illness, or affect the well being of workers. These hazards or stressors are typically divided into the categories biological, chemical, physical, ergonomic and psychosocial. The risk of a health effect from a given stressor is a function of the hazard multiplied by the exposure to the individual or group. For chemicals, the hazard can be understood by the dose response profile most often based on toxicological studies or models. Occupational hygienists work closely with toxicologists for understanding chemical hazards, physicists for physical hazards, and physicians and microbiologists for biological hazards. Environmental and occupational hygienists are considered experts in exposure science and exposure risk management. Depending on an individual's type of job, a hygienist will apply their exposure science expertise for the protection of workers, consumers and/or communities.

The British Occupational Hygiene Society (BOHS) defines that "occupational hygiene is about the prevention of ill-health from work, through recognizing, evaluating and controlling the risks". The International Occupational Hygiene Association (IOHA) refers to occupational hygiene as *the discipline of anticipating, recognizing, evaluating and controlling health hazards in the working environment with the objective of protecting worker health and well-being and safeguarding the community at large.* The term "occupational hygiene" (used in the UK and Commonwealth countries as well as much of Europe) is synonymous with *industrial hygiene* (used in the US, Latin America, and other countries that received initial technical support or training from US sources). The term "industrial hygiene" traditionally stems from industries with construction, mining or manufacturing and "occupational hygiene" refers to all types of industry such as those listed for "industrial hygiene" as well as financial and support services industries and refers to "work", "workplace" and "place of work" in general. *Environmental hygiene* addresses similar issues to *occupational hygiene*, but is likely to be about broad industry or broad issues affecting the local community, broader society, region or country.

The profession of occupational hygiene uses strict and rigorous scientific methodology and often requires professional judgment based on experience and education in determining the potential for hazardous exposure risks in workplace and environmental studies. These aspects of occupational hygiene can often be referred to as the "art" of occupational hygiene and is used in a similar sense to the "art" of medicine. In fact "occupational hygiene" is both an aspect of preventative medicine and in particular occupational medicine, in that its goal is to prevent industrial disease, using the science of risk management, exposure assessment and industrial safety. Ultimately professionals seek to implement "safe" systems, procedures or methods to be applied in the workplace or to the environment.

The Social Role of Occupational Hygiene

Occupational hygienists have been involved historically with changing the perception of society about the nature and extent of hazards and preventing exposures in the workplace and communities. Many occupational hygienists work day-to-day with industrial situations that require control or improvement to the workplace situation however larger social issues affecting whole industries have occurred in the past e.g. since 1900, asbestos exposures that have affected the lives of tens of thousands of people. Occupational hygienists have become more engaged in understanding and managing exposure risks to consumers from products with new regulations such as REACh (Registration, Evaluation, Authorisation and Restriction of Chemicals).

More recent issues affecting broader society are, for example in 1976, legionnaires' disease or legionellosis. More recently again in the 1990s radon and in the 2000s the effects of mold from indoor air quality situations in the home and at work. In the later part of the 2000s concern has been raised about the health effects of nanoparticles.

Many of these issues have required the coordination over a number of years of a number of medical and para professionals in detecting and then characterizing the nature of the issue, both in terms of the hazard and in terms of the risk to the workplace and ultimately to society. This has involved occupational hygienists in research, collection of data and to develop suitable and satisfactory control methodologies.

General Activities

The occupational hygienist may be involved with the assessment and control of physical, chemical, biological or environmental hazards in the workplace or community that could cause injury or disease. Physical hazards may include noise, temperature extremes, illumination extremes, ionizing or non-ionizing radiation, and ergonomics. Chemical hazards related to dangerous goods or hazardous substances are frequently investigated by occupational hygienists. Other related areas including indoor air quality (IAQ) and safety may also receive the attention of the occupational hygienist. Biological hazards may stem from the potential for legionella exposure at work or the investigation of biological injury or effects at work, such as dermatitis may be investigated.

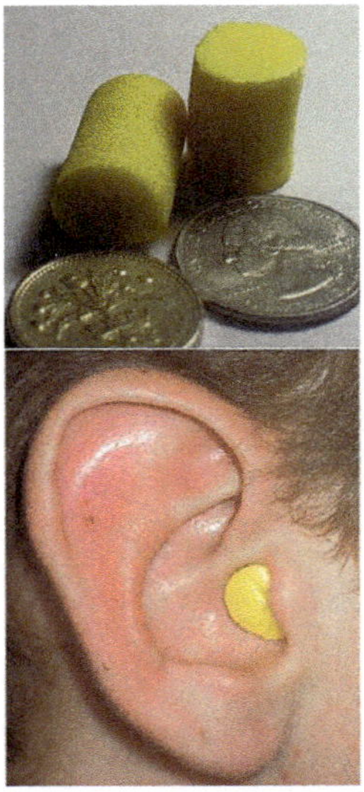

Disposable foam earplugs: out of the ear with coins for scale (top)
and inserted into the wearer's ear (bottom).

As part of the investigation process, the occupational hygienist may be called upon to communicate effectively regarding the nature of the hazard, the potential for risk, and the appropriate methods of control. Appropriate controls are selected from the hierarchy of control: by elimination, substitution, engineering, administration and personal protective equipment (PPE) to control the hazard or eliminate the risk. Such controls may involve recommendations as simple as appropriate PPE such as a 'basic' particulate dust mask to occasionally designing dust extraction ventilation systems, work places or management systems to manage people and programs for the preservation of health and well-being of those who enter a workplace.

Examples of occupational hygiene include:

- Analysis of physical hazards such as noise that would lead to use of earplugs or earmuffs.
- Planning procedures to protect against infectious disease exposure in the event of a flu pandemic.
- Monitoring and testing the air for hazardous contaminants that can lead to potential worker illness and/or death.

Workplace Assessment Methods

Although there are many aspects to occupational hygiene work the most known and sought after is in determining or estimating potential or actual exposures to hazards. For many chemicals and physical hazards, occupational exposure limits have been derived using toxicological, epidemiological and medical data allowing hygienists to reduce the risks of health effects by implementing the "Hierarchy of Hazard Controls". Several methods can be applied in assessing the workplace or environment for exposure to a known or suspected hazard. Occupational hygienists do not rely on the accuracy of the equipment or method used but in knowing with certainty and precision the limits of the equipment or method being used and the error or variance given by using that particular equipment or method. Well known methods for performing occupational exposure assessments can be found in "A Strategy for Assessing and Managing Occupational Exposures, Third Edition Edited by Joselito S. Ignacio and William H. Bullock".

The main steps outlined for assessing and managing occupational exposures:

- Basic Characterization (identify agents, hazards, people potentially exposed and existing exposure controls)
- Exposure Assessment (select occupational exposure limits, hazard bands, relevant toxicological data to determine if exposures are "acceptable", "unacceptable" or "uncertain")
- Exposure Controls (for "unacceptable" or "uncertain" exposures)
- Further Information Gathering (for "uncertain" exposures)
- Hazard Communication (for all exposures)
- Reassessment (as needed) / Management of Change

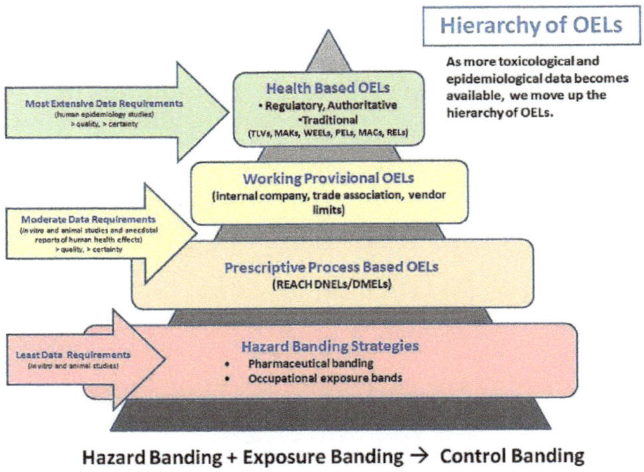

Hierarchy of occupational exposure limits (OELs)

Basic Characterization, Hazard Identification and Walk-through Surveys

The first step in understanding health risks related to exposures requires the collection of "basic characterization" information from available sources. A traditional method applied by occupational hygienists to initially survey a workplace or environment is used to determine both the types and possible exposures from hazards (e.g. noise, chemicals, radiation). The walk-through survey can be targeted or limited to particular hazards such as silica dust, or noise, to focus attention on control of all hazards to workers. A full walk-through survey is frequently used to provide information on establishing a framework for future investigations, prioritizing hazards, determining the requirements for measurement and establishing some immediate control of potential exposures. The Health Hazard Evaluation Program from the National Institute for Occupational Safety and Health is an example of an industrial hygiene walk-through survey. Other sources of basic characterization information include worker interviews, observing exposure tasks, material safety data sheets, workforce scheduling, production data, equipment and maintenance schedules to identify potential exposure agents and people possibly exposed.

The information that needs to be gathered from sources should apply to the specific type of work from which the hazards can come from. As mentioned previously, examples of these sources include interviews with people who have worked in the field of the hazard, history and analysis of past incidents, and official reports of work and the hazards encountered. Of these, the personnel interviews may be the most critical in identifying undocumented practices, events, releases, hazards and other relevant information. Once the information is gathered from a collection of sources, it is recommended for these to be digitally archived (to allow for quick searching) and to have a physical set of the same information in order for it to be more accessible. One innovative way to display the complex historical hazard information is with a historical hazards identification map, which distills the hazard information into an easy to use graphical format.

Sampling

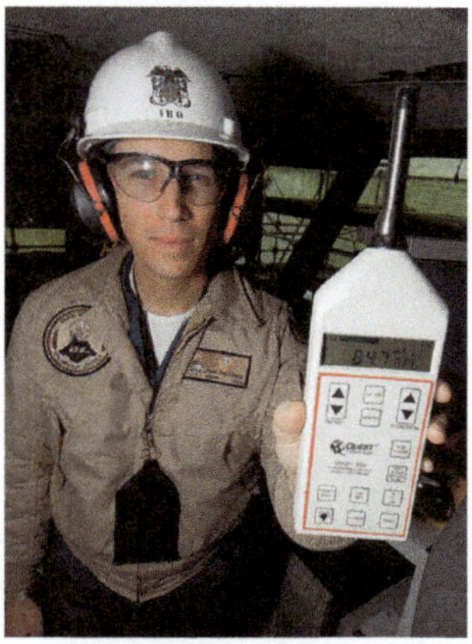

Measurements of noise levels using a sound level meter is a component of the occupational hygiene assessment.

An occupational hygienist may use one or a number of commercially available electronic measuring devices to measure noise, vibration, ionizing and non-ionizing radiation, dust, solvents, gases, and so on. Each device is often specifically designed to measure a specific or particular type of contaminant. Such devices are often subject to multiple interferences. Electronic devices need to be calibrated before and after use to ensure the accuracy of the measurements taken and often require a system of certifying the precision of the instrument.

Dust Sampling

Nuisance dust is considered to be the total dust in air including inhalable and respirable fractions.

Various dust sampling methods exist that are internationally recognised. Inhalable dust is determined using the modern equivalent of the Institute of Occupational Medicine (IOM) MRE 113A monitor. Inhalable dust is considered to be dust of less than 100 micrometers aerodynamic equivalent diameter (AED) that enters through the nose and or mouth.

Respirable dust is sampled using a cyclone dust sampler design to sample for a specific fraction of dust AED at a set flow rate. The respirable dust fraction is dust that enters the 'deep lung' and is considered to be less than 10 micrometers AED.

Nuisance, inhalable and respirable dust fractions are all sampled using a constant volumetric pump for a specific sampling period. By knowing the mass of the sample collected and the volume of air sampled a concentration for the fraction sampled can be given in milligrams (mg) per metre cubed (m3). From such samples the amount of inhalable or respirable dust can be determined and compared to the relevant occupational exposure limits.

By use of inhalable, respirable or other suitable sampler (7 hole, 5 hole, et cetera) these dust sampling methods can also used to determine metal exposure in the air. This requires collection of the sample on a methyl-cellulose ester (MCE) filter and acid digestion of the collection media in the laboratory followed by measuring metal concentration though an atomic absorption (or emission) spectrophotometery. Both the UK Health and Safety Laboratory and NIOSH Manual of Analytical Methods have specific methodologies for a broad range of metals in air found in industrial processing (smelting, foundries, et cetera).

A further method exists for the determination of asbestos, fibreglass, synthetic mineral fibre and ceramic mineral fibre dust in air. This is the membrane filter method (MFM) and requires the collection of the dust on a grided filter for estimation of exposure by the counting of 'conforming' fibres in 100 fields through a microscope. Results are quantified on the basis of number of fibres per millilitre of air (f/ml). Many countries strictly regulate the methodology applied to the MFM.

Chemical Sampling

Two types of chemically absorbent tubes are used to sample for a wide range of chemical substances. Traditionally a chemical absorbent 'tube' (a glass or stainless steel tube of between 2 and 10 mm internal diameter) filled with very fine absorbent silica (hydrophilic) or carbon, such as coconut charcoal (lypophylic), is used in a sampling line where air is drawn through the absorbent material for between four hours (minimum workplace sample) to 24 hours (environmental sample) period. The hydrophilic material readily absorbs water-soluble chemical and the lypophylic material absorbs non water-soluble materials. The absorbent material is then chemically or physically extracted and measurements performed using various gas chromatograph or mass spectrometry methods. These absorbent tube methods have the advantage of being usable for a wide range of potential contaminates. However, they are relatively expensive methods, are time consuming and require significant expertise in sampling and chemical analysis. A frequent complaint of workers is in having to wear the sampling pump (up to 1 kg) for several days of work to provide adequate data for the required statistical certainty determination of the exposure.

In the last few decades, advances have been made in 'passive' badge technology. These samplers can now be purchased to measure one chemical (e.g. formaldehyde) or a chemical type (e.g. ketones) or a broad spectrum of chemicals (e.g. solvents). They are relatively easy to set up and use. However, considerable cost can still be incurred in analysis of the 'badge'. They weigh 20 to 30 grams and workers do not complain about their presence. Unfortunately 'badges' may not exist for all types of workplace sampling that may be required and the charcoal or silica method may sometimes have to be applied.

From the sampling method, results are expressed in milligrams per cubic meter (mg/m3) or parts per million (PPM) and compared to the relevant occupational exposure limits.

It is a critical part of the exposure determination that the method of sampling for the specific contaminate exposure is directly linked to the exposure standard used. Many countries regulate both the exposure standard, the method used to determine the exposure and the methods to be used for chemical or other analysis of the samples collected.

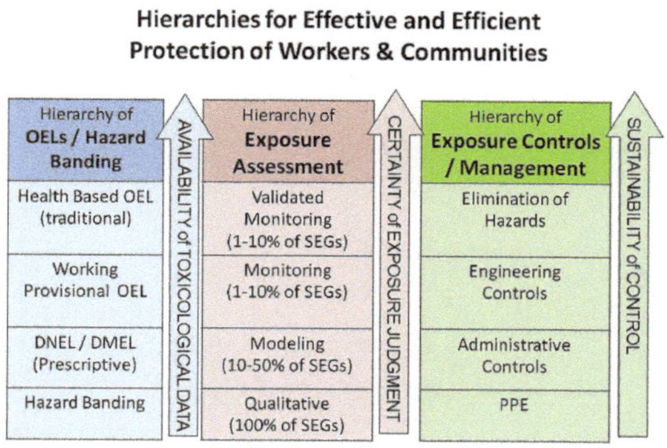

Simple representation of exposure risk assessment and management hierarchy based on available information

Exposure Management and Controls

The hierarchy of control defines the approach used to reduce exposure risks protecting workers and communities. These methods include elimination, substitution, engineering controls (isolation or ventilation), administrative controls and personal protective equipment. Occupational hygienists, engineers, maintenance, management and employees should all be consulted for selecting and designing the most effective and efficient controls based on the hierarchy of control.

Professional Societies

The development of industrial hygiene societies originated in the United States, beginning with the first convening of members for the American Conference of Governmental Industrial Hygienists in 1938, and the formation of the American Industrial Hygiene Association in 1939. In the United Kingdom, the British Occupational Hygiene Society started in 1953. Through the years, professional occupational societies have formed in many different countries, leading to the formation of the International Occupational Hygiene Association in 1987, in order to promote and develop occupational hygiene worldwide through the member organizations. The IOHA has grown to 29 member organizations, representing over 20,000 occupational hygienists worldwide, with representation from countries present in every continent.

Peer-reviewed Literature

There are several academic journals specifically focused on publishing studies and research in the occupational health field. The *Journal of Occupational and Environmental Hygiene* (JOEH) has been published jointly since 2004 by the American Industrial Hygiene Association and the American Conference of Governmental Industrial Hygienists, replacing the former *American Industrial Hygiene Association Journal* and *Applied Occupational & Environmental Hygiene* journals. Another seminal occupational hygiene journal would be *The Annals of Occuapational Hygiene,* published by the British Occupational Hygiene Society since 1958. Further, The National Institute for Occupational Safety and Health maintains a searchable bibliographic database (NIOSHTIC-2) of occupational safety and health publications, documents, grant reports, and other communication products.

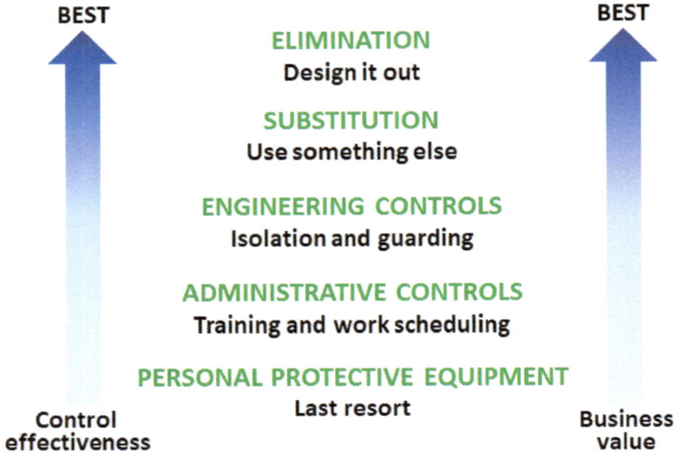
BEST
BEST
ELIMINATION
Design it out
SUBSTITUTION
Use something else
ENGINEERING CONTROLS
Isolation and guarding
ADMINISTRATIVE CONTROLS
Training and work scheduling
PERSONAL PROTECTIVE EQUIPMENT
Last resort
Control effectiveness
Business value

The hierarchy of controls is an important tool to determine hEducationow to control hazards most efficiently and effectively in a workplace.

Occupational Hygiene as a Career

Examples of occupational hygiene careers include:

- Compliance officer on behalf of regulatory agency
- Professional working on behalf of company for the protection of the workforce
- Consultant working on behalf of companies
- Researcher performing laboratory or field occupational hygiene work

Education

The basis of the technical knowledge of occupational hygiene is from competent training in the following areas of science and management.

- Basic Sciences (Biology, Chemistry, Mathematics (Statistics), Physics);
- Occupational Diseases (Illness, injury and health surveillance (biostatistics, epidemiology, toxicology));

- Health Hazards (Biological, Chemical and Physical hazards, Ergonomics and Human Factors);
- Working Environments (Mining, Industrial, Manufacturing, transport and storage, service industries and offices);
- Programme Management Principles (professional and business ethics, work site and incident investigation methods, exposure guidelines, Occupational exposure limits, jurisdictional based regulations, hazard identification, risk assessment and risk communication, data management, fire evacuation and other emergency responses);
- Sampling, measurement and evaluation practices (instrumentation, sampling protocols, methods or techniques, analytical chemistry);
- Hazard Controls (elimination, substitution, engineering, administrative, PPE and Air Conditioning and Extraction Ventilation);
- Environment (air pollution, hazardous waste).

However, it is not rote knowledge that identifies a competent occupational hygienist. There is an "art" to applying the technical principles in a manner that provides a reasonable solution for workplace and environmental issues. In effect an experienced "mentor", who has experience in occupational hygiene is required to show a new occupational hygienist how to apply the learned scientific and management knowledge in the workplace and to the environment issue to satisfactorily resolve the problem.

To be a professional occupational hygienist, experience in as wide a practice as possible is required to demonstrate knowledge in areas of occupational hygiene. This is difficult for "specialists" or those who practice in narrow subject areas. Limiting experience to individual subject like asbestos remediation, confined spaces, indoor air quality, or lead abatement, or learning only through a textbook or "review course" can be a disadvantage when required to demonstrate competence in other areas of occupational hygiene.

Information can be considered to be only an outline of the requirements for professional occupational hygiene training. This is because the actual requirements in any country, state or region may vary due to educational resources available, industry demand or regulatory mandated requirements.

During 2010, the Occupational Hygiene Training Association (OHTA) through sponsorship provided by the IOHA initiated a training scheme for those with an interest in or those requiring training in occupational hygiene. These training modules can be downloaded and used freely. The available subject modules (Basic Principles in Occupational Hygiene, Health Effects of Hazardous Substances, Measurement of Hazardous Substances, Thermal Environment, Noise, Asbestos, Control, Ergonomics) are aimed at the 'foundation' and 'intermediate' levels in Occupational Hygiene. Although the modules can be used freely without supervision attendance at an accredited training course is encouraged. These training modules are available from OH Learning.com

Academic programs offering industrial hygiene bachelor's or master's degrees in United States may apply to the Accreditation Board for Engineering and Technology (ABET) to have their program accredited. As of October 1, 2006, 27 institutions have accredited their industrial hygiene programs. Accreditation is not available for Doctoral programs.

In the U.S. the training of IH professionals is supported by National Institute for Occupational Safety and Health through their NIOSH Education and Research Centers.

Professional Credentials

Australia

In 2005, the Australian Institute of Occupational Hygiene (AIOH) has accredited professional occupational hygienist through a certification scheme. Occupational Hygienists in Australian certified through this scheme are entitled to use the phrase Certified Occupational Hygienist (COH) as part of their qualifications.

United States of America

Practitioners who successfully meet specific education and work-experience requirements, and pass a written examination administered by the American Board of Industrial Hygiene (ABIH) are authorized to use the term Certified Industrial Hygienist (CIH) or Certified Associate Industrial Hygienist (CAIH). Both of these terms have been codified into law in many states in the United States to identify minimum qualifications of individuals having oversight over certain activities that may affect employee and general public health.

After the initial certification, the CIH or CAIH maintains their certification by meeting on-going requirements for ethical behavior, education, and professional activities (e.g., active practice, technical committees, publishing, teaching).

ABIH certification examinations are offered during a spring and fall testing window each year at more than 400 locations worldwide.

The CIH designation is the most well known and recognized industrial hygiene designation throughout the world. There are approximately 6800 CIHs in the world making ABIH the largest industrial hygiene certification organization. The CAIH certification program was discontinued in 2006. Those who were certified as a CAIH retain their certification through ongoing certification maintenance. People who are currently certified by the ABIH can be found in a public roster.

The ABIH is a recognized certification board by the International Occupational Hygiene Association (IOHA). The CIH certification has been accredited internationally by the International Organization for Standardization/International Electrotechnical

Commission (ISO/IEC 17024). In the United States, the CIH has been accredited by the Council of Engineering and Scientific Specialty Boards [CESB].

The Association of Professional Industrial Hygienists, Inc. (APIH) was established in 1994 to offer credentialing to industrial hygienists who meet the education and experience requirements found in Tennessee Code Annotated, Title 62, Chapter 40. APIH adopted the Tennessee Code as its basis for credentialing because it was the first legal definition in the United States of an industrial hygienist in terms of education and experience. The APIH Registration Committee investigates and verifies, through electronic means or correspondence, both educational and experience accomplishments claimed by each applicant for registration. The Committee determines the appropriate level of registration, Registered Industrial Hygienist or Registered Professional Industrial Hygienist, and then authorizes the registration certificate to be issued.

Canada

In Canada, a practitioner who successfully completes a written and an interview administered by the Canadian Registration Board of Occupational Hygienists can be recognized as a Registered Occupational Hygienist (ROH) or Registered Occupational Hygiene Technician (ROHT). There is also designation to be recognized as a Canadian Registered Safety Professional (CRSP).

United Kingdom

The Faculty of Occupational Hygiene, part of the British Occupational Hygiene Society, represents the interests of professional occupational hygienists.

Membership of the Faculty of Occupational Hygiene is confined to BOHS members who hold a recognized professional qualification in occupational hygiene.

There are three grades of Faculty membership:

- Licentiate (LFOH) holders will have obtained the BOHS Certificate of Operational Competence in Occupational Hygiene and have at least three years' practical experience in the field.
- Members (MFOH) are normally holders of the Diploma of Professional Competence in Occupational Hygiene and have at least five years' experience at a senior level.
- Fellows (FFOH) are senior members of the profession who have made a distinct contribution to the advancement of occupational hygiene.

All Faculty members participate in a Continuous Professional Development (CPD) scheme designed to maintain a high level of current awareness and knowledge in occupational hygiene.

India

Indian Society of Industrial hygiene was formed in 1981 at Chennai India. Subsequently, its secretariat was shifted to Kanpur. The society has registered about 400 members, about 90 of whom life members. The society publishes a newsletter "Industrial Hygiene Link". The current address of the secretary of the society is Shyam Singh Gautam, Secretary, Indian Society of Industrial Hygiene, 11, Shakti Nagar, Rama Devi, Kanpur 2008005 Mobile number 8005187037.

References

- "NIOSH Pocket Guide to Chemical Hazards" (PDF). Centers for Disease Control and Prevention. September 2007. Retrieved June 29, 2016
- Editorial. (2006). "Nanomedicine: A matter of rhetoric?". Nat Materials. 5 (4): 243. PMID 16582920. doi:10.1038/nmat1625
- Abrams, Herbert K. (2001). "A Short History of Occupational Health" (PDF). Journal of Public Health Policy. 22 (1): 34–80. PMID 11382089. doi:10.2307/3343553. Retrieved 9 August 2012
- "Current Intelligence Bulletin 63: Occupational Exposure to Titanium Dioxide" (PDF). United States National Institute for Occupational Safety and Health. Retrieved 2012-02-19
- Wagner V, Dullaart A, Bock AK, Zweck A (2006). "The emerging nanomedicine landscape". Nat. Biotechnol. 24 (10): 1211–1217. PMID 17033654. doi:10.1038/nbt1006-1211
- Chaturvedi, Pradeep (2006-01-01). Challenges of Occupational Safety and Health: Thrust : Safety in Transportation. Concept Publishing Company. ISBN 9788180692840
- Smith, Erin Geiger (14 February 2013). "U.S.-based inventors lead world in nanotechnology patents: study". Technology. Reuters. Retrieved 4 June 2016
- Shaffer RE, Rengasamy S (2009). "Respiratory protection against airborne nanoparticles: a review". J Nanopart Res. 11: 1661–1672. doi:10.1007/s11051-009-9649-3
- Stephan, Constantin (2012), Industrial Health, Safety and Environmental Management, epubli, Berlin, 3rd edition 2012, ISBN 978-3-7418-7478-9, pp. 70-71
- Hale A, Ytehus I, 2004, 'Changing requirements for the safety profession: roles and tasks', Journal of Occupational Health & Safety – Australia and New Zealand
- "Guidance note: General duty of care in Western Australian workplaces 2005" (PDF). Government of Western Australia. Retrieved 15 July 2014
- Rengasamy S, Eimer BC (2011). "Total inward leakage of nanoparticles through filtering facepiece respirators". Ann Occup Hyg. 55: 253–263. doi:10.1093/annhyg/meq096
- Churcher D W, Alwani-Starr G M,Incorporating construction health and safety into the design process", Implementation of Health and Safety in Construction Sites, Alvels, Dias & Coble (eds), ISBN 90-5410-847-9, 1996
- Keenan, A., & Newton, T.J. (1985). Stressful events, stressors and psychological strains in young professional engineers. Journal of Occupational Behaviour, 6(2), 151-156. doi:10.1002/job.4030060206
- "Construction Safety and Health". Workplace Safety & Health Topics. National Institute of Occupational Safety and Health. Retrieved 3 August 2012

- Kuhlbusch T, et al. (2011). "Nanoparticle exposure at nanotechnology workplaces: a review". Part. Fibre Toxicol. 8 (1): 22. doi:10.1186/1743-8977-8-22
- O'Brien, James J. (2013-04-17). Construction Inspection Handbook: Quality Assurance/Quality Control. Springer Science & Business Media. ISBN 9781475711912
- Hashemi, L., & Webster, B.S. (1998). Non-fatal workplace violence workers' compensation claims (1993 1996). Journal of Occupational and Environmental Medicine, 40, 561-567. doi:10.1016/S0749-3797(03)00095-3
- Phillips, Owen (30 June 2017). "The USPS is an extremely dangerous place to work". The Outline (website). Retrieved 30 June 2017
- Trist, E.L., & Bamforth, K.W. (1951). Some social and psychological consequences of the longwall method of coal getting. Human Relations, 14, 3-38. doi:10.1177/001872675100400101
- Das, Siddhartha (6 June 2015). "Occupational fatalities in the construction sector: A medico-legal viewpoint". Medicolegal Journal. 83: 93–97. doi:10.1177/0025817214554869
- "Risks and nanotechnology: the public is more concerned than experts and industry" (PDF). Nature Publishing Group. 2007. Retrieved 20 March 2013
- Zohar, D. (2010). Thirty years of safety climate research: Reflections and future directions. Accident Analysis and Prevention, 42, 1517-1522. doi: 10.1016/j.aap.2009.12.019

4

Physical Ergonomics

Occupational diseases are diseases that occur in humans because of their occupational activity. Some examples of known occupational diseases are lung diseases, skin diseases, etc. Occupational injuries are injuries sustained in the workplace, especially while carrying out hazardous work. The topics elaborated in this chapter will help in gaining a better perspective about physical ergonomics.

Occupational Disease

An occupational disease is any chronic ailment that occurs as a result of work or occupational activity. It is an aspect of occupational safety and health. An occupational disease is typically identified when it is shown that it is more prevalent in a given body of workers than in the general population, or in other worker populations. The first such disease to be recognised, squamous-cell carcinoma of the scrotum, was identified in chimney sweep boys by Sir Percival Pott in 1775. Occupational hazards that are of a traumatic nature (such as falls by roofers) are not considered to be occupational diseases.

Under the law of workers' compensation in many jurisdictions, there is a presumption that specific disease are caused by the worker being in the work environment and the burden is on the employer or insurer to show that the disease came about from another cause. Diseases compensated by national workers compensation authorities are often termed occupational diseases. However, many countries do not offer compensations for certain diseases like musculoskeletal disorders caused by work (e.g. in Norway). Therefore, the term work-related diseases is utilized to describe diseases of occupational origin. This term however would then include both compensable and non-compensable diseases that have occupational origins.

Examples

Some well-known occupational diseases include:

Lung Diseases

Occupational lung diseases include asbestosis among asbestos miners and those who work with friable asbestos insulation, as well as black lung (coalworker's pneumoconiosis) among coal miners, silicosis among miners and quarrying and tunnel operators and byssinosis among workers in parts of the cotton textile industry.

Occupational asthma has a vast number of occupations at risk.

Bad indoor air quality may predispose for diseases in the lungs as well as in other parts of the body.

Skin Diseases

Occupational skin diseases are ranked among the top five occupational diseases in many countries.

Occupational skin diseases and conditions are generally caused by chemicals and having wet hands for long periods while at work. Eczema is by far the most common, but urticaria, sunburn and skin cancer are also of concern.

Contact dermatitis due to irritation is inflammation of the skin which results from a contact with an irritant. It has been observed that this type of dermatitis does not require prior sensitization of the immune system. There have been studies to support that past or present atopic dermatitis is a risk factor for this type of dermatitis. Common irritants include detergents, acids, alkalies, oils, organic solvents and reducing agents.

The acute form of this dermatitis develops on exposure of the skin to a strong irritant or caustic chemical. This exposure can occur as a result of accident at a workplace . The irritant reaction starts to increase in its intensity within minutes to hours of exposure to the irritant and reaches its peak quickly. After the reaction has reached its peak level, it starts to heal. This process is known as decrescendo phenomenon. The most frequent potent irritants leading to this type of dermatitis are acids and alkaline solutions. The symptoms include redness and swelling of the skin along with the formation of blisters.

The chronic form occurs as a result of repeated exposure of the skin to weak irritants over long periods of time.

Clinical manifestations of the contact dermatitis are also modified by external factors such as environmental factors (mechanical pressure, temperature, and humidity) and predisposing characteristics of the individual (age, sex, ethnic origin, preexisting skin disease, atopic skin diathesis, and anatomic region exposed.

Another occupational skin disease is Glove related hand urticaria. It has been reported as an occupational problem among the health care workers. This type of hand urticaria is believed to be caused by repeated wearing and removal of the gloves. The reaction is caused by the latex or the nitrile present in the gloves.

High-risk occupations include:

- Hairdressing
- Catering

- Healthcare
- Printing
- Metal machining
- Motor vehicle repair
- Construction

Other Diseases of Concern

- Overuse syndrome among persons who perform repetitive or forceful movements in constrictive postures
- Carpal tunnel syndrome among persons who work in the poultry industry and information technology
- Computer vision syndrome among persons using information technology for hours
- Lead poisoning affecting workers in many industries that processed or employed lead or lead compounds

Historical

Donald Hunter in his classic history of occupational diseases discusses many example of occupational diseases. They include:

- Phossy jaw among the London matchgirls
- Radiation sickness among some persons who had been working in the nuclear industry
- Radium jaw among the Radium Girls
- Squamous cell carcinoma of the skin of the scrotum among chimney sweeps (Chimney sweeps' carcinoma)

Prevention

Prevention measures include avoidance of the irritant through its removal from the workplace or through technical shielding by the use of potent irritants in closed systems or automation, irritant replacement or removal and personal protection of the workers.

In order to better prevent and control occupational disease, most countries revise and update their related laws, most of them greatly increasing the penalties in case of breaches of the occupational disease laws. Occupational disease prevention, in general legally regulated, is part of good supply chain management and enables companies to design and ensure supply chain social compliance schemes as well as monitor their implementation to identify and prevent occupational disease hazards.

Occupational Lung Disease

Occupational lung diseases are occupational diseases affecting the respiratory system, including occupational asthma, black lung disease (coalworker's pneumoconiosis), chronic obstructive pulmonary disease (COPD), mesothelioma, and silicosis. Infectious lung diseases can also be acquired in an occupational context. Exposure to substances like flock and silica can cause fibrosing lung disease, whereas exposure to carcinogens like asbestos and beryllium can cause lung cancer. Occupational cases of interstitial lung disease may be misdiagnosed as COPD, idiopathic pulmonary fibrosis, or a myriad of other diseases; leading to a delay in identification of the causative agent.

Types of Occupational Lung Diseases

Asbestosis

Asbestosis is a fibrosing interstitial lung disease caused by exposure to forms of the mineral asbestos.

Asthma

Asthma is a respiratory disease that can begin or worsen due to exposure at work and is characterized by episodic narrowing of the respiratory tract. Occupational asthma has a variety of causes, including sensitization to a specific substance, causing an allergic response; or a reaction to an irritant that is inhaled in the workplace. Exposure to various substances can also worsen pre-existing asthma. People who work in isocyanate manufacturing, who use latex gloves, or who work in an indoor office environment are at higher risk for occupational asthma than the average US worker. Approximately 2 million people in the US have occupational asthma.

Coalworker's Pneumoconiosis (Black Lung)

Coalworker's pneumoconiosis, also called "black lung disease", is an interstitial lung disease caused by long-term exposure (over 10 years) to coal dust. Symptoms include shortness of breath and lowered pulmonary function. It can be fatal when advanced. Between 1970-1974, prevalence of CWP among US coal miners who had worked over 25 years was 32%; the same group saw a prevalence of 9% in 2005-2006.

COPD

Chronic obstructive pulmonary disease is a respiratory disease that can encompass chronic bronchitis and/or emphysema. 15% of the cases of COPD in the United States can be attributed to occupational exposure, including exposure to silica and coal dust. People who work in mining, construction, manufacturing (specifically textiles, rubber, plastic, and leather), building, and utilities are at higher risk for COPD than the average US worker.

Indium Lung

Indium lung is an interstitial lung disease caused by occupational exposure to indium tin oxide.

Mesothelioma

Mesothelioma is a cancer of the mesothelium, part of which is the pleura, the lining of the lungs. Mesothelioma is caused by exposure to asbestos.

Silo-filler's Disease

Silo-Filler's disease results from inhalation of nitrogen dioxide (NO_2) gas from fresh silage. The presentation is variable depending on level of exposure. Often the gas penetrates throughout the lung and if severe can manifest as a form of Acute Respiratory Distress Syndrome, such as significant pulmonary edema, hyalinized alveolar membranes, congestion and other respiratory illnesses.

Silicosis

Silicosis is a fibrosing interstitial lung disease caused by inhaling fine particles of silica, most commonly in the form of quartz or cristobalite. Short-term exposures of large amounts of silica or long-term (10 years or more) exposure of lower levels of silica can cause silicosis. In 1968, more than 1060 US workers died of silicosis; this number fell to 170 by 2005.

World Trade Center Lung

World Trade Center lung is a cluster of diseases caused by exposure to fallout at Ground Zero of the September 11 attacks in 2001. These diseases include asthma, asthmatic bronchitis, terminal airways disease, sarcoidosis, and acute eosinophilic pneumonia.

Occupational Environmental Exposure

Arsenic

Arsenic is classified as an IARC Group 1 carcinogen and is a cause of lung cancer. Workers can be exposed to arsenic through work with some pesticides or in copper smelting.

Asbestos

Asbestos is a mineral which was extensively used in the United States to fireproof buildings and textiles, among other items, in the 1950s-1980s. Workers are frequently exposed to asbestos during demolition and renovation work, which can cause asbestosis and/or mesothelioma. Asbestos exposure can also cause pleural effusion, diffuse pleural fibrosis, pleural plaques, and non-mesothelioma lung cancer. Smoking greatly increases the lung cancer risk of asbestos exposure.

BCME

BCME (Bis(chloromethyl) ether) is associated with small cell lung cancer in workers who have been exposed. Exposure can occur via direct manufacture of BCME or its presence as a byproduct.

Beryllium

Beryllium is classified as an IARC Group 1 carcinogen and is used in a wide variety of industries. Those who are manufacturing workers, dental technicians, machinists, jewelers, plumbers, electricians, precious metal reclamation workers, and welders are at risk for beryllium exposure.

Cadmium

Cadmium is classified as an IARC Group 1 carcinogen and it is a cause of several cancers, including lung cancer. Workers can be exposed to cadmium through welding, zinc smelting, copper smelting, lead smelting, electroplating, battery manufacture, plastics manufacture, and in alloying.

Chromium

Chromium is classified as an IARC Group 1 carcinogen and is linked to lung cancer. Workers can be exposed to chromium via welding, steel manufacturing, pigment/dye manufacturing, and electroplating.

Coal Dust

Exposure to coal dust is the cause of coalworker's pneumoconiosis. It can also exacerbate or cause COPD.

Diesel Exhaust

Diesel exhaust contains a variety of gaseous and particulate chemicals, including soot, polycyclic aromatic hydrocarbons, and other known carcinogens.

Flock

Flocking is the technique of adding small pieces of nylon or other material to a backing, usually a textile, to create a contrasting texture. Inhalation of flock can cause flock worker's lung.

Nanoparticles

The high surface area to volume ratio of nanoparticles may make them an inhalation hazard for workers exposed to them. This is a topic of ongoing research as of 2015.

Nickel

Nickel is classified by the IARC as a Group 1 carcinogen; nickel compound exposure is associated with nasal cancer as well as lung cancer. Workers may be exposed to nickel in machining/grinding industry, nickel extraction/production, welding, and electroplating.

Polycyclic Aromatic Hydrocarbons

Polycyclic aromatic hydrocarbons (PAHs), fused-ring chemicals formed during the combustion of fossil fuels, are metabolized by the cytochrome P450 complex to highly reactive carbocations, which can mutate DNA and cause cancer. Workers may be exposed to PAHs while working in a foundry, in the roofing industry, or due to environmental tobacco smoke.

Silica

Besides causing silicosis, inhalation of silica can cause or exacerbate COPD. It can also impair lung function in general and cause cancer by oxidation damage. It is classified as a "known human carcinogen" (Group 1 carcinogen) by the IARC. Exposure is common for people working in tunneling, quarrying, construction, sandblasting, roadway repair, mining, and foundry work.

Tobacco Smoke

Tobacco smoke is a known carcinogen. Workers in the hospitality industry may be exposed to tobacco smoke in the workplace, especially in environments like casinos and bars/restaurants.

Infectious Exposure

Influenza

Health care professionals are at risk of occupational influenza exposure; during a pandemic influenza, anyone in a close environment is at risk, including those in an office environment.

Tuberculosis

Tuberculosis is a lung disease endemic in many parts of the world. Health care professionals and prison guards are at high risk for occupational exposure to tuberculosis, since they work with populations with high rates of the disease.

Occupational Asthma

Occupational asthma is an occupational lung disease and a type of asthma. Like other types of asthma, it is characterized by airway inflammation, reversible airways obstruction, and bronchospasm, but it is caused by something in the workplace environment.

Symptoms include shortness of breath, tightness of the chest, nasal irritation, coughing and wheezing. The first person to use it in reference to a medical condition was Hippocrates, and he believed that tailors, anglers and metalworkers were more likely to be affected by the disease. Although much research has been done since, the inflammatory component of asthma was recognized only in the 1960s.

Hypersensitivity pneumonitis is a related condition, with many occupational examples (e.g. flock worker's lung, farmer's lung, and indium lung). However, although overlapping in many cases, hypersensitivity pneumonitis may be distinguished from occupational asthma in that it isn't restricted to only occupational exposure, and involves type III hypersensitivity and type IV hypersensitivity rather than the type I hypersensitivity of asthma. Also, unlike asthma, hypersensitivity pneumonitis targets lung alveoli rather than bronchi.

Signs and Symptoms

Less than five years of exposure or a single exposure to a high-concentration agent can result in symptoms. Coughing, wheezing, nasal irritation, shortness of breath, and chest tightness are the most common symptoms, all of which worsen after work and improve during time away from work. Pre-existing asthma can be exacerbated by similar agents.

Risk Factors

At present, over 400 workplace substances have been identified as having asthmagenic or allergenic properties. Their existence and magnitude vary by region and industry and can include diisocyanates, acid anhydrides, plicatic acid, and platinum salts (all low molecular weight agents), and animal protein, enzymes, wheat, and latex (high-molecular weight agents). For example, in France the industries most affected are bakeries and cake-shops, automobile industry and hairdressers, whereas in Canada the principal cause is wood dust, followed by isocyanates. Furthermore, the most common cause of occupational asthma in the workplace are isocyanates. Isocyanates are used in the production of motor vehicles and in the application of orthopaedic polyurethane and fibreglass casts.

The occupations most at risk are: adhesive handlers (e.g. acrylate), animal handlers and veterinarians (animal proteins), bakers and millers (cereal grains), carpet makers (gums), electronics workers (soldering resin), forest workers, carpenters and cabinetmakers (wood dust), hairdressers (e.g. persulfate), health care workers (latex and chemicals such as glutaraldehyde), janitors and cleaning staff (e.g. chloramine-T), pharmaceutical workers (drugs, enzymes), seafood processors, shellac handlers (e.g. amines), solderers and refiners (metals), spray painters, insulation installers, plastics and foam industry workers (e.g. diisocyanates), textile workers (dyes) and users of plastics and epoxy resins (e.g. anhydrides)

Diagnosis

Diagnosis of occupational asthma uses several techniques.

A non-specific bronchial hyperreactivity test can be used to help diagnose occupational asthma. It involves testing with methacoline, after which the forced expiratory volume in 1 second (FEV_1) of the patient is measured. This test is often used for measuring the intensity of a person's asthma and to confirm that the person needs to be treated for asthma.

Other non specific tests could require the patient to run for a few minutes at a continuous pace. In this case, the individual's peak expiratory flow rate (PEFR) is measured, showing how fast a person can exhale. PEFR can also be measured at work to see if there is a difference from the PEFR in a controlled environment. Measuring PEFR at work is a highly reliable test for occupational asthma.

A skin prick test is usually performed on the inner forearm where a grid is marked and a drop of the allergens to be tested are placed on the arm in the grid. Once this has been done, the skin is pricked through the drop using a lancet. Reactions, if any, occur within 10 to 15 minutes and these results can then be analyzed.

Immunoglobulin E is an antibody found in human blood and is effective against toxins. Since it can also trigger allergic reactions to specific allergens like pollen, the IgE test is performed to evaluate whether the subject is allergic to these substances.

A spirometer is a device used to measure timed expired and inspired volumes, and can be used to help diagnose occupational asthma.

Specific inhalation challenges test for reactions to substances found in the workplace. One method is a whole body sealed chamber where the patient is exposed to articles that are present in their workplace. This method has the advantage of being able to assess, albeit highly subjectively, ocular and nasal symptoms as well as a reduction in FEV_1. Another test requires the patient to breathe aerosols of the suspected asthmagens through an oro-facial mask. These asthmagens are aerosolized using closed circuit chambers, and the quantities and concentrations administered are minute and extremely stable, to minimize the risk of exaggerated responses.

Prevention

Prevention of occupational asthma can be accomplished through better education of workers, management, unions and medical professionals. This will enable them to identify the risk factors and put in place preventive measures, including respiratory protection and exposure limits.

Treatment

Recovery is directly dependent on the duration and level of exposure to the causative agent. Depending on the severity of the case, the condition of the patient can improve dramatically during the first year after removal from exposure.

Three basic types of procedures are used for treating the affected workers: reducing a worker's exposure, removing a worker from the environment with the asthma-causing agent, and treatment with asthma medications. Completely stopping exposure is more effective treatment than reducing exposure. By reducing exposure, the probability of suffering another reaction is lowered. Methods of reducing exposure include transferring an affected worker to a position without the relevant asthmagen, use of respiratory protection, and engineering controls. In 1984 innovator David Cornell discovered and invented effective control equipment in the UK for the removal of many harmful workplace fumes. 'BOFA' extraction products are now found in over 100 countries worldwide.

People affected by occupational asthma that occurred after a latency period, whether a few months or years, should be immediately removed from exposure to the causative agent. However, this can entail severe socio-economic consequences for the worker as well as the employer due to loss of job, unemployment, compensation issues, quasi-permanent medical expenditures, and hiring and re-training of new personnel. This can be mitigated by transferring the worker within a company.

Medication

Short-acting beta-agonists like salbutamol or terbutaline or long-acting beta-agonists like salmeterol and formoterol dilate airways which relieve the symptoms thus reducing the severity of the reaction. Some patients also use it just before work to avoid a drop in the FEV_1.

Anti-inflammatory agents like corticosteroids, LKTRA or mast cell stabilizers can also be used depending on the severity of the case.

Epidemiology

Approximately 21% of the adults affected by asthma report an aggravation of their symptoms while at work and an improvement when away, which implies that they may be suffering from occupational asthma. In the United States, occupational asthma is the most common occupational lung disease. Today, asthma affects as much as 15% of the Canadian population, a statistic reflective of other developed countries, and has increased fourfold in the last 20 years. Various reasons can be identified for this increase, including increase environmental pollution, better diagnostic ability, and greater awareness.

Society and Culture

Compensation

When a person is diagnosed with occupational asthma, it can result in serious socio-economic consequences not only for the workers but also for the employer and the healthcare system because the worker must change positions. The probability of being re-employed is lower for those with occupational asthma compared to those with normal asthma. The employer not only pays compensation to the employee, but will also have to spend a considerable amount of time and energy and funds for hiring and training new personnel. In the United States, it was estimated that the direct cost of occupational asthma in 1996 was $1.2 billion and the indirect cost $0.4 billion, for a total cost of $1.6 billion.

Occupational Stress

Occupational stress is stress related to one's job. Occupational stress often stems from unexpected responsibilities and pressures that do not align with a person's knowledge, skills, or expectations, inhibiting one's ability to cope. Occupational stress can increase when workers do not feel supported by supervisors or colleagues, or feel as if they have little control over work processes.

Models

Because stress results from the complex interactions between a large system of interrelated variables, there are several psychological theories and models that address occupational stress.

Person Environment Fit Model: This model "suggests that the match between a person and their work environment is key in influencing their health. For healthy conditions, it is necessary that employees' attitudes, skills, abilities and resources match the demands of their job, and that work environments should meet workers' needs, knowledge, and skills potential. Lack of fit in either of these domains can cause problems, and the greater the gap or misfit (either subjective or objective) between the person and their environment, the greater the strain as demands exceed abilities, and need exceeds supply. These strains can relate to health related issues, lower productivity, and other work problems. Defense mechanisms, such as denial, reappraisal of needs, and coping, also operate in the model, to try and reduce subjective misfit"

Job Characteristics Model: This model "focuses on important aspects of job characteristics, such as skill variety, task identity, task significance, autonomy, and feedback. These characteristics are proposed to lead to 'critical psychological states' of experienced meaningfulness, and experienced responsibility and knowledge of outcomes. It is proposed that positive or negative work characteristics give rise to mental states which lead to corresponding cognitive and behavioral outcomes, e.g. motivation, satisfaction, absenteeism, etc. In conjunction with the model, Hackman and Oldham (1980) developed the Job Diagnostic Survey, a questionnaire for job analysis, which implies key types of job-redesign including combining tasks, creating feedback methods, job enrichment, etc."

Diathesis-Stress Model: This model looks at behaviors as a susceptibility burden together with stress from life experiences. It is useful to distinguish stressful job conditions or stressors from an individual's reactions or strains. Strains can be mental, physical or emotional. Occupational stress can occur when there is a discrepancy between the demands of the environment/workplace and an individual's ability to carry out and complete these demands. Often a stressor can lead the body to have a physiological reaction that can strain a person physically as well as mentally. A variety of factors contribute to workplace stress such as excessive workload, isolation, extensive hours worked, toxic work environments, lack of autonomy, difficult relationships among coworkers and management, management bullying, harassment and lack of opportunities or motivation to advancement in one's skill level.

Jobs-Demand Resources Model: This model posits that strain are a response to imbalance between demands of one's job and the resources he or she has to deal with those demands.

- Job demands: the physical, psychological, social, or organizational aspects of a job that require sustained physical and/or psychological effort or skills. Therefore, they are associated with expenditure of time and energy.
- Job resources: the physical, psychological, social, or organizational aspects of the job that aid in achieving work goals; reduce job demands and the associated physiological and psychological cost; stimulate personal growth, learning, and development.

Effort-Reward Imbalance Model: This model focuses on the reciprocal relationship between efforts and rewards at work. "More specifically, the ERI Model claims that work characterized by both high efforts and low rewards represents a reciprocity deficit between high 'costs' and low 'gains', which could elicit negative emotions in exposed employees. The accompanying feelings may cause sustained strain reactions. So, working hard without receiving adequate appreciation or being treated fairly are examples of a stressful imbalance. Another assumption of the ERI Model concerns individual differences in the experience of effort-reward imbalance. It is assumed that employees characterized by a motivational pattern of excessive job-related commitment and a high need for approval (i.e., overcommitment) will respond with more strain reactions to an effort-reward imbalance, in comparison with less overcommitted people."

Sources of occupational stress come from:

- a toxic work environment
- negative workload
- isolation
- types of hours worked
- role conflict & role ambiguity
- lack of autonomy, career development barriers
- difficult relationships with administrators and/or coworkers
- managerial bullying
- towing to the wrong gates
- harassment,
- and organizational climate.

These individual sources demonstrate that stress can occur specifically when a conflict arises from the job demands of the employee and the employee itself. If not handled properly, the stress can become distress.

1. Coping: the ability of the employee coping with the specific hours worked, the level of productive rate expected, the physical environment, as well as the expectancy of the work desired by management. For instance, research shows that night shifts in particular has a high possibility of negative impact towards the health of the employee. In relation to this, approximately 20 percent of night shift workers have experienced psycho-physiological dysfunctions, including heart diseases. Extreme factors can affect the competence levels of employees.

2. Role in the organization: associated with the hierarchical ranking of that particular employee within the organization. Upper management is entitled to oversee the overall functioning of the organization. This causes potential distress as the employee must be able to perform simultaneous tasks.

3. Career development: Security of their occupation, promotion levels, etc. are all sources of stress, as this business market in terms of technology of economic dominance is ever-changing.

4. Interpersonal relationships within the workplace: The workplace is a communication and interaction based industry. These relationships (either developed or developing) can be problematic or positive. Common stressors include harassment, discrimination, biased opinions, hearsay, and other derogatory remarks.

5. Organizational climate or structure: The overall communication, management style, and participation among groups of employees are variables to be considered. In essence, the resultant influence of the high participation rate, collaborative planning, and equally dispersed responsibilities provides a positive effect on stress reduction, improved work performance, job satisfaction, and decreased psychosomatic disorders.

Prevalence

Distress is a prevalent and costly problem in today's workplace. About one-third of workers report high levels of stress. 20-30% of workers in different sectors of the European Union reported in 2007 that they believed work-related stress was potentially affecting their health. Three-quarters of employees believe the worker has more on-the-job stress than a generation ago. In Great Britain, a sixth of the workforce experiences occupational stress every year. Evidence also suggests that distress is the major cause of turnover in organizations. With continued distress at the workplace, workers will develop psychological and physiological dysfunctions and decreased motivation in excelling in their position. Increased levels of job stress are determined by the awareness of having little control but lots of demands in the work area. Occupational stress and its sequelae represent the majority of work-related illnesses causing missed work days. Those in the protective services, transportation and materials moving, building grounds cleaning and maintenance, and healthcare are more susceptible to both work injuries and illnesses, as well as work-related stress.

Negative Health Effects

Stress-related disorders encompass a broad array of conditions, including psychological disorders (e.g., depression, anxiety, post-traumatic stress disorder) and other types of emotional strain (e.g., dissatisfaction, fatigue, tension, etc.), maladaptive behaviors (e.g., aggression, substance abuse), and cognitive impairment (e.g., concentration and memory problems). In turn, these conditions may lead to poor work performance, higher absenteeism, less work productivity or even injury. "If untreated, consistently high stress can become a chronic condition, which can exacerbate existing mental health conditions and chronic physical conditions (diabetes, hypertension, weak immune system). These conditions not only diminish the well-being of workers and increase the employer's health benefits expenses, they contribute to increased injury incidence. Consistently high levels of stress increase the risk of occupational injury. A study of light/short haul truckers, a group that experiences high rates of injury and mental health issues, found that frequent stress increased the odds of occupational injury by 350%."

Job stress is also associated with various biological reactions that may lead ultimately to compromised health, such as cardiovascular disease, or in extreme cases death. Due to the high pressure and demands in the work place the demands have been shown to be correlated with increased rates of heart attack, hypertension and other disorders. In New York, Los Angeles, and London, among other municipalities, the relationship between job stress and heart attacks is acknowledged.

Problems at work are more strongly associated with health complaints than are any other life stressor-more so than even financial problems or family problems. Occupational stress accounts for more than 10% of work-related health claims. Many studies suggest that psychologically demanding jobs that allow employees little control over the work process increase the risk of cardiovascular disease. Research indicates that job stress increases the risk for development of back and upper-extremity musculoskeletal disorders. Other disorders that can be caused or exacerbated by occupational stress include sleep disorders, headache, mood disorders, upset stomach, hypertension, high cholesterol, autoimmune disease, cardiovascular disease, depression, and anxiety. Stress at work can also increase the risk of acquiring an infection and the risk of accidents at work.

High levels of stress are associated with substantial increases in health service utilization. Workers who report experiencing stress at work also show excessive health care utilization. In a 1998 study of 46,000 workers, health care costs were nearly 50% greater for workers reporting high levels of stress in comparison to "low risk" workers. The increment rose to nearly 150%, an increase of more than $1,700 per person annually, for workers reporting high levels of both stress and depression. Health care costs increase by 200% in those with depression and high occupational stress. Additionally, periods of disability due to job stress tend to be much longer than disability periods for other occupational injuries and illnesses.

Physiological reactions to stress can have consequences for health over time. Researchers have been studying how stress affects the cardiovascular system, as well as how work stress can lead to hypertension and coronary artery disease. These diseases, along with other stress-induced illnesses tend to be quite common in American work-places. There are four main physiological reactions to stress:

- Blood is shunted to the brain and large muscle groups, and away from extremities, skin, and organs that are not currently serving the body.
- An area near the brain stem, known as the reticular activating system, goes to work, causing a state of keen alertness as well as sharpening of hearing and vision.

- Energy-providing compounds of glucose and fatty acids are released into the bloodstream.
- The immune and digestive systems are temporarily shut down.

Gender

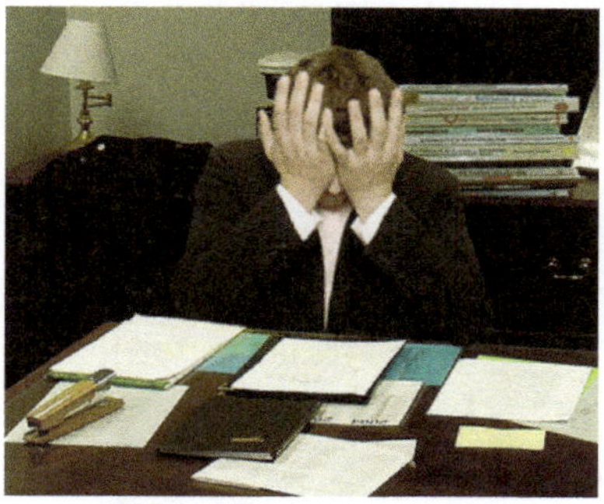

Frustrated man at a desk

Men and women are exposed to many of the same stressors. Although men and women might not differ in overall strains, women are more likely to experience psychological distress, whereas men experience more physical strain. Desmarais and Alksnis suggest two explanations for the greater psychological distress of women. First, the genders may differ in their awareness of negative feelings, leading women to express and report strains, whereas men deny and inhibit such feelings. Second, the demands to balance work and family result in more overall stressors for women that leads to increased strain.

The Kenexa Research Institute released a global survey of almost 30,000 workers which showed that females suffered more workplace distress than their male counterparts. According to the survey, women's stress level were 10% higher for those in supervisory positions, 8% higher stress in service and production jobs than men, and 6% higher in middle and upper management than men in the same position.

Causes

Job stress results from various interactions of the worker and the environment of the work they perform their duties. Location, gender, environment, and many other factors contribute to the buildup of stress. Job stress results from the interaction of the worker and the conditions of work. Views differ on the importance of worker characteristics versus working conditions as the primary cause of job stress. The differing viewpoints suggest different ways to prevent stress at work. Differences in individual characteristics such as personality and coping skills can be very important in predicting whether certain job conditions will result in stress. In other words, what is stressful for one person may not be a problem for someone else. This viewpoint underlies prevention strategies that focus on workers and ways to help them cope with demanding job conditions. In general, occupational stress is caused by a mismatch between perceived effort and perceived reward, and/or a sense of low control in a job with high demands. Low social support at work and job insecurity can also increase occupational stress. Psychosocial stressors are a major cause of occupational stress.

Working Conditions

Although the importance of individual differences cannot be ignored, scientific evidence suggests that certain working conditions are stressful to most people. Such evidence argues for a greater emphasis on working conditions as the key source of job stress, and for job redesign as a primary prevention strategy. Large surveys of working conditions, including conditions recognized as risk factors for job stress, were conducted in member states of the European Union in 1990, 1995, and 2000. Results showed a time trend suggesting an increase in work intensity. In 1990, the percentage of workers reporting that they worked at high speeds at least one-quarter of their working time was 48%, increasing to 54% in 1995 and to 56% in 2000. Similarly, 50% of workers reported they work against tight deadlines at least one-fourth of their working time in 1990, increasing to 56% in 1995 and 60% in 2000. However, no change was noted in the period 1995–2000 (data not collected in 1990) in the percentage of workers reporting sufficient time to complete tasks.

Workload

In an occupational setting, dealing with workload can be stressful and serve as a stressor for employees. There are three aspects of workload that can be stressful.

- Quantitative workload or overload: Having more work to do than can be accomplished comfortably.
- Qualitative workload: Having work that is too difficult.
- Underload: Having work that fails to use a worker's skills and abilities.

Workload as a work demand is a major component of the demand-control model of stress. This model suggests that jobs with high demands can be stressful, especially when the individual has low control over the job. In other words, control serves as a buffer or protective factor when demands or workload is high. This model was expanded into the demand-control-support model that suggests that the combination of high control and high social support at work buffers the effects of high demands.

As a work demand, workload is also relevant to the job demands-resources model of stress that suggests that jobs are stressful when demands (e.g., workload) exceed the individual's resources to deal with them.

Long Hours

A substantial percentage of Americans work very long hours. By one estimate, more than 26% of men and more than 11% of women worked 50 hours per week or more in

2000. These figures represent a considerable increase over the previous three decades, especially for women. According to the Department of Labor, there have been a rise in increasing amount of hours in the work place by employed women, an increase in extended work weeks (>40 hours) by men, and a considerable increase in combined working hours among working couples, particularly couples with young children.

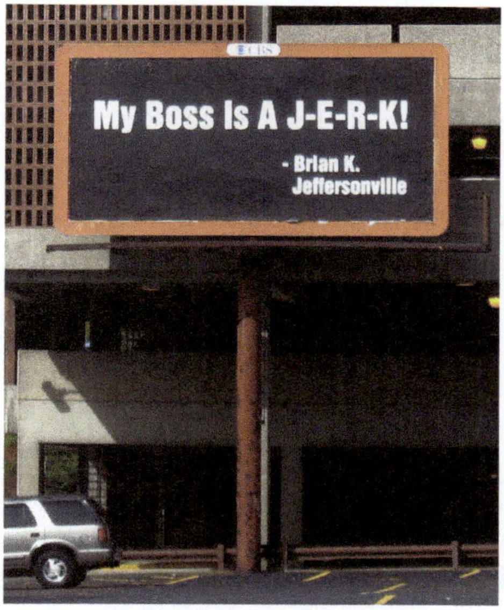

Evidence of occupational stress due to an individual's status in the workplace

Status

A person's status in the workplace can also affect levels of stress. While workplace stress has the potential to affect employees of all categories; those who have very little influence to those who make major decisions for the company. However, less powerful employees (that is, those who have less control over their jobs) are more likely to suffer stress than powerful workers. Managers as well as other kinds of workers are vulnerable to work overload.

Economic Factors

Economic factors that employees are facing in the 21st century have been linked to increased stress levels. Researchers and social commentators have pointed out that the computer and communications revolutions have made companies more efficient and productive than ever before. This boon in productivity however, has caused higher expectations and greater competition, putting more stress on the employee.

The following economic factors may lead to workplace stress:

- Pressure from investors, who can quickly withdraw their money from company stocks.

- The lack of trade and professional unions in the workplace.
- Inter-company rivalries caused by the efforts of companies to compete globally
- The willingness of companies to swiftly lay off workers to cope with changing business environments.

Bullying

Bullying in the workplace can also contribute to stress. This can be broken down into five different categories:

- Threat to profession status
- Threat to personal status
- Isolation
- Excess work
- Destabilization i.e. lack of credit for work, meaningless tasks etc.

This in effect can create a hostile work environment for the employees that, which in turn, can affect their work ethic and contribution to the organization.

Narcissism and Psychopathy

Thomas suggests that there tends to be a higher level of stress with people who work or interact with a narcissist, which in turn increases absenteeism and staff turnover. Boddy finds the same dynamic where there is corporate psychopath in the organisation.

Workplace Conflict

Interpersonal conflict among people at work has been shown to be one of the most frequently noted stressors for employees. Conflict has been noted to be an indicator of the broader concept of workplace harassment. It relates to other stressors that might co-occur, such as role conflict, role ambiguity, and workload. It also relates to strains such as anxiety, depression, physical symptoms, and low levels of job satisfaction.

Sexual Harassment

Women are more likely than men to experience sexual harassment, especially for those working in traditionally masculine occupations. In addition, a study indicated that sexual harassment negatively affects workers' psychological well-being. Another study found that level of harassment at workplaces lead to differences in performance of work related tasks. High levels of harassment were related to the worst outcomes, and no harassment was related to least negative outcomes. In other words, women who had experienced a higher level of harassment were more likely to perform poorly at workplaces.

Occupational Group

Lower occupational groups are at higher risk of work-related ill health than higher occupational groups. This is in part due to adverse work and employment conditions. Furthermore, such conditions have greater effects on ill-health to those in lower socio-economic positions.

Effects

Stressful working conditions can lead to three types of strains: Behavioral (e.g., absenteeism or poor performance), physical (e.g., headaches or coronary heart disease), and psychological (e.g., anxiety or depressed mood). Physical symptoms that may occur because of occupational stress include fatigue, headache, upset stomach, muscular aches and pains, weight gain or loss, chronic mild illness, and sleep disturbances. Psychological and behavioral problems that may develop include anxiety, irritability, alcohol and drug use, feeling powerless and low morale. The spectrum of effects caused by occupational stress includes absenteeism, poor decision making, lack of creativity, accidents, organizational breakdown or even sabotage. If exposure to stressors in the workplace is prolonged, then chronic health problems can occur including stroke. An examination was of physical and psychological effects of workplace stress was conducted with a sample of 552 female blue collar employees of a microelectronics facility. It was found that job-related conflicts were associated with depressive symptoms, severe headaches, fatigue, rashes, and other multiple symptoms. Studies among the Japanese population specifically showed a more than 2-fold increase in the risk of total stroke among men with job strain (combination of high job demand and low job control). Those in blue-collar or maual labor jobs are more likely to develop heart disease compared to those in white-collar jobs. Along with the risk of stroke, stress can raise the risk of high blood pressure, immune system dysfunction, coronary artery disease. Prolonged occupational stress can lead to occupational burnout. Occupational stress can also disrupt relationships.

The effects of job stress on chronic diseases are more difficult to ascertain because chronic diseases develop over relatively long periods of time and are influenced by many factors other than stress. Nonetheless, there is some evidence that stress plays a role in the development of several types of chronic health problems—including cardiovascular disease, musculoskeletal disorders, and psychological disorders. Job stress and strain has been associated with poor mental health and wellbeing over a 12-year period.

Occupational stress has negative effects for organizations and employers. Occupational stress is the cause of approximately 40% of turnover and 50% of workplace absences. The annual cost of occupational stress and its effects in the US is estimated to be over $60 billion to employers and $250–300 billion to the economy.

Prevention

A combination of organizational change and stress management is often the most useful approach for preventing stress at work. Both organizations and employees can employ strategies at organizational and individual levels. Generally, organizational level strategies include job procedure modification and employee assistance programs (EAP). Individual level strategies include taking vacation. Getting a realistic job preview to understand the normal workload and schedules of the job will also help people to identify whether or not the job fit them.

How an Organization Can Prevent Job Stress

- Ensure that the workload is in line with workers' capabilities and resources.
- Design jobs to provide meaning, stimulation, and opportunities for workers to use their skills.
- Clearly define workers' roles and responsibilities.
- To reduce workplace stress, managers may monitor the workload given out to the employees. Also while they are being trained they should let employees understand and be notified of stress awareness.
- Give workers opportunities to participate in decisions and actions affecting their jobs.
- Improve communications-reduce uncertainty about career development and future employment prospects.
- Provide opportunities for social interaction among workers.
- Establish work schedules that are compatible with demands and responsibilities outside the job.
- Combat workplace discrimination (based on race, gender, national origin, religion or language).
- Bringing in an objective outsider such as a consultant to suggest a fresh approach to persistent problems.
- Introducing a participative leadership style to involve as many subordinates as possible to resolve stress-producing problems.
- Encourage work-life balance through family-friendly benefits and policies

An insurance company conducted several studies on the effects of stress prevention programs in hospital settings. Program activities included (1) employee and management education on job stress, (2) changes in hospital policies and procedures to reduce organizational sources of stress, and (3) the establishment of employee assistance programs. In one study, the frequency of medication errors declined by 50% after prevention activities were implemented in a 700-bed hospital. In a second study, there was a 70% reduction in malpractice claims in 22 hospitals that implemented stress prevention activities. In contrast, there was no reduction in claims in a matched group of 22 hospitals that did not implement stress prevention activities.

Telecommuting is another way organizations can help reduce stress for their workers. Employees defined telecommuting as "an alternative work arrangement in which employees perform tasks elsewhere that are normally done in a primary or central workplace, for at least some portion of their work schedule, using electronic media to interact with others inside and outside the organization." One reason that telecommuting gets such high marks is that it allows employees more control over how they do their work. Telecommuters reported more job satisfaction and less desire to find a new job. Employees that worked from home also had less stress, improved work/life balance and higher performance rating by their managers.

A systematic review of stress-reduction techniques among healthcare workers found that cognitive behavioral training lowered emotional exhaustion and feelings of lack of personal accomplishment.

Signs and Symptoms of Excessive Job and Workplace Stress

Signs and symptoms of excessive job and workplace stress include:

• Feeling anxious, irritable, or depressed	• Muscle tension or headaches
• Apathy, loss of interest in work	• Stomach problems
• Problems sleeping	• Social withdrawal
• Fatigue	• Loss of sex drive
• Trouble concentrating	• Using alcohol or drugs to cope

Both yoga and mindful-based stress reduction have been shown to reduce work-related stress. Nursings participating in cognitive behavioral interventions less perceived stress, a greater sense of coherence, and increased mood.

Expanding Research on Stress: Contemporary opinions hold that jobs designed to support skill variety, task identity, significance, autonomy, and feedback, while providing for existence and growth needs, will sustain a healthier, greater satisfied workforce.

For team-oriented work environments, Patrick Lencioni's The Five Dysfunctions of a Team profiles the behavior of cohesive teams:

1. They trust one another

2. They engage in unfiltered conflict around ideas

3. They commit to decisions and plans of action
4. They hold one another accountable for delivering against those plans
5. They focus on the achievement of collective results.

For immediate individual stress management, rudimentary mental coping strategies may be adopted in the work environment.

Occupational Injury

An occupational injury is bodily damage resulting from working. The most common organs involved are the spine, hands, the head, lungs, eyes, skeleton, and skin. Occupational injuries can result from exposure to occupational hazards (physical, chemical, biological, or psychosocial), such as temperature, noise, insect or animal bites, blood-borne pathogens, aerosols, hazardous chemicals, radiation, and occupational burnout.

While many prevention methods are set in place, injuries may still occur due to poor ergonomics, manual handling of heavy loads, misuse or failure of equipment, exposure to general hazards, and inadequate safety training.

Worldwide

It has been estimated that worldwide there are more than 350,000 workplace fatalities and more than 270 million workplace injuries annually. In 2000 there were approximately 2.9 billion workers worldwide. Occupational injuries resulted in the loss of 3.5 years of healthy life for every 1,000 workers. 300,000 of the occupational injuries resulted in a fatality.

The most common occupations associated with these hazards vary throughout the world depending on the major industries in a particular country. Overall, the most hazardous occupations are in farming, fishing, and forestry. In more developed countries, construction and manufacturing occupations are associated with high rates of spine, hand, and wrist injuries.

United States

In the United States in 2012, 4,383 workers died from job injuries, 92% of which were men, and nearly 3 million nonfatal workplace injuries & illness were reported which cost businesses a collective loss of $198.2 billion and 60 million workdays. In 2007, 5,488 workers died from job injuries, 92% of which were men, and 49,000 died from work-related injuries. NIOSH estimates that 4 million workers in the U.S. in 2007 suffered from non-fatal work related injuries or illnesses.

According to data from the National Institute for Occupational Safety and Health (NIOSH) and the Bureau of Labor Statistics, an average of 15 workers die from traumatic injuries each day in the United States, and an additional 200 workers are hospitalized.

In a study in the state of Washington, injured workers were followed for 14 years to determine the long term effects of work injury on employment. The work injuries resulted in an average of 1.06 years of lost productivity for each of the 31,588 allowed claims.

Dangerous Sectors

In the U.S. the Bureau of Labor Statistics makes available extensive statistics on workplace accidents and injuries. For example:

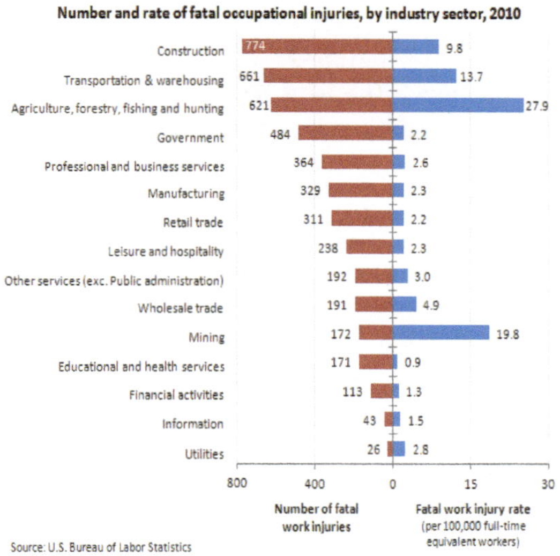

Common Injuries

As in the United Kingdom, slips, trips and falls are common and account for 20-40% of disabling occupational injuries. Often these accidents result in a back injury that can persist to a permanent disability. In the United States, a high risk of back injuries occurs in the health care industry. 25% of reported injuries in health care workers in the state of Pennsylvania are for back pain. Among nurses, the prevalence of lower back pain may be as high as 72% mostly as a result of transferring patients. Fortunately, some of these injuries can be prevented with the availability of patient lifts, improved worker training, and allocation of more time to perform work procedures. Another common type of injury is carpal tunnel syndrome associated with overuse of the hands and wrists. Studies on a cohort of newly hired workers have thus far identified forceful gripping, repetitive lifting of > 1 kg, and using vibrating power tools as high risk work activities.

Additionally, noise exposure in the workplace can cause hearing loss, which accounted for 14% of reported occupational illnesses in 2007. Many initiatives have been created to prevent this common workplace injury. For example, the Buy Quiet program encourages employers to purchase tools and machines that produce less noise and the Safe-In-Sound Award was created to recognize companies and program that excel in the area of hearing loss prevention.

Accidental injection or needlestick injuries are a common injury that plague agriculture workers and veterinarians. The majority of these injuries are located to the hands or legs, and can result in mild to severe reactions, including possible hospitalization. Due to the wide variety of biologics used in animal agriculture, needlestick injuries can result in bacterial or fungal infections, lacerations, local inflammation, vaccine/antibiotic reactions, amputations, miscarriage, and death. Due to daily human-animal interactions, livestock related injuries are also a prevalent injury of agriculture workers, and are responsible for the majoriy of nonfatal worker injuries on dairy farms. Additionally, approximately 30 people die of cattle and horse-related deaths in the United States annually.

Employees at Risk

Perhaps the most important personal factor that predisposes to an increased risk is age. In the United States in 1998 17 million workers were over age 55 and by 2018 this population is expected to more than double. Workers in this age group are more likely to suffer from lower back pain that may be worsened by work conditions that normally do not affect a younger worker. Older workers are also more likely by be killed in a construction related fall. They are also at higher risk for injury due to age-related hearing loss, visual impairment, and use of multiple prescription medications that has been linked to higher rates of work injuries. In addition to age, other personal risk factors for injury include obesity particularly its associated risk with back injury, and depression.

Lack of proper education or training can also predispose an individual to an occupational injury. For example, there is limited needlestick injury awareness among agriculture workers, and there is a need for comprehensive programs to prevent needlestick injuries on livestock operations. Proper animal handling techniques and training, or stockmanship, can also decrease the risk of livestock injury. A handler's timing, positioning, speed, direction of movement, and sounds made will affect the behavior of an animal and consequently the safety of the handler. The agriculture industry has begun to focus more on proper education and training, and has made a variety of resources available to producers. For example, organizations like the Upper Midwest Agriculture Safety and Health Center (UMASH) have a variety of informational fact sheets and training videos easily accessible online. Additionally, organizations like Beef Quality Assurance offers stockmanship training seminars and demonstrations.

Regulation

In the United States, the Occupational Safety and Health Administration (OSHA) sets and enforces national standards for occupational safety across all sectors.

United Kingdom

In the United Kingdom in 2013/2014, 133 people were killed at work. Of those 133 people, 89 were employed, while 44 were self-employed. In 2013/2014, an estimated 629,000 injuries occurred at work. Of these injuries 629,000 injuries, 203,000 led to more than 3 days absence from work. Of these, over 148,000 resulted in the victim being absent from work for more than 7 days.

Dangerous Sectors

- Construction: 42 deaths
- Agriculture: 27 deaths
- Waste and Recycling: four deaths
- Other: 60 deaths

Of all the workplace accidents that resulted in death, the most common were falls from height, contact with moving machinery and being struck by a vehicle. These types of accidents resulted in over half of all recorded deaths.

Common Injuries

Slips, trips and falls account for over a third of all injuries that happen at work. Incorrect handling of items was the most common cause of injuries that led to absences from work of more than 7 days. Upper limb injuries represented 47.3% of workplace injuries in 2010-2011, the most common area injured.

In all, over 1,900,000 working days were lost in 2013/2014 due to slips, trips and falls.

Employer Prosecutions

The Health & Safety Executive (HSE) prosecuted 582 cases in 2013/2014, with at least one conviction secured in 547 cases (94%).

Local authorities prosecuted a total of 92 cases during the same period, with at least one conviction achieved in 89 cases (97%).

A total of 13,790 notices were issued by the HSE and local authorities, with over £16,700,000 issued in fines.

Employees at Risk

Unsurprisingly, occupation is the biggest influence on the risk of workplace injuries. Workers new to the job are at a much higher risk of injury than more experienced staff, while shift workers and part-time staff also have a greater risk of being injured at work.

Taiwan

In Taiwan, there were 14,261 occupational injuries recorded in 2010. 45% of these involved trauma to the upper limbs.

Prevention

There are many methods of preventing or reducing industrial injuries, including anticipation of problems by risk assessment, safety training, control banding, personal protective equipment safety guards, mechanisms on machinery, and safety barriers. In addition, past problems can be analyzed to find their root causes by using a technique called root cause analysis. A 2013 Cochrane review found low-quality evidence showing that inspections, especially focused inspections, can reduce work-related injuries in the long term.

References

- Chan-Yeung, Moira; Malo, Jean-Luc (1995). "Occupational Asthma". New England Journal of Medicine. 333 (2): 107–112. ISSN 0028-4793. PMID 7777015. doi:10.1056/NEJM199507133330207
- "NIOSH Work Organization and Stress Related Disorders". United States National Institute for Occupational Safety and Health. Retrieved 2007-12-01
- Mohr LC (September 2004). "Hypersensitivity pneumonitis". Curr Opin Pulm Med. 10 (5): 401–11. PMID 15316440. doi:10.1097/01.mcp.0000135675.95674.29
- Colligan, Thomas W; Colligan MSW; Higgins M. (2006). "Workplace Stress - Etiology and Consequences" (PDF). Journal of Workplace Behavioral Health. 21 (2): 89–97. doi:10.1300/J490v21n02_07
- Safety, Government of Canada, Canadian Centre for Occupational Health and. "Dermatitis, Irritant Contact : OSH Answers". www.ccohs.ca. Retrieved 2016-03-25

- Liu, C.; Spector, P. E.; Shi, L. (2007). "Cross-National Job Stress: A Quantitative and Qualitative Study". Journal of Organizational Behavior. 28 (2): 209–239. doi:10.1002/job.435
- Page 503 in: Mitchell, Richard Sheppard; Kumar, Vinay; Abbas, Abul K.; Fausto, Nelson (2007). Robbins Basic Pathology. Philadelphia: Saunders. ISBN 1-4160-2973-7. 8th edition
- Buswell, ML.; Hourigan, M. (2015). "Needlestick Injuries in Agriculture Workers and Prevention Programs". Journal of Agromedicine. 21 (1). PMID 26478987. doi:10.1080/1059924X.2015.1106996. Retrieved 1 August 2016
- "Bis(chloromethyl)ether (BCME) (CASRN 542-88-1)". IRIS (Integrated Risk Information System). EPA. 31 October 2014. Retrieved 31 March 2015
- Karasek, R. A. (1979). "Job demands, job decision latitude, and mental strain-implications for job redesign". Administrative Science Quarterly. 24 (2): 285–308. doi:10.2307/2392498
- Gyllensten, K. (2005). "The role of gender in workplace stress: A critical literature review". Health Education Journal. 64 (64 (3)): 271–288. doi:10.1177/001789690506400307
- "Ten Years of Working Conditions in the European Union, 2005". European Foundation for the Improvement of Living and Working Conditions. Retrieved 2007-12-01
- Gajendran, Ravi; Harrison, David (2008). "Telecommuting Win-Win For Employees And Employers". Journal of Applied Psychology. 92 (6): 5–5. doi:10.1037/0021-9010.92.6.1524
- Farrow, A.; Reynolds, F. (2012-01-01). "Health and safety of the older worker". Occupational Medicine. 62 (1): 4–11. ISSN 1471-8405. PMID 22201131. doi:10.1093/occmed/kqr148

5

Diverse Aspects of Occupational Ergonomics

The diverse aspects of occupational ergonomics are Rohmert's law, engineering psychology, workplace aggression, etc. Any type of aggression which occurs in the workplace is known as workplace aggression. The behavior ranges from verbal abuses to degrading a person to physical abuse. This chapter has been carefully written to provide an easy understanding of the diverse aspects of occupational ergonomics.

Rohmert's Law

Widely used in the human factors and ergonomics field, Rohmert's law states that the maximum force one's muscles can exert decreases exponentially from the time one begins continuously exerting the force. It is commonly used to calculate "maximum holding time" for any particular task.

Maximum force decays exponentially due to the amount of energy (in the form of oxygen and ATP) the body is able to supply to the muscles. The circulatory systems keeps muscles flooded in nutrients at all times, so that muscles have a supply of fuel ready to burn at any given moment. A task requiring maximum force burns a large amount of those nutrients at the onset of the task; the circulatory system is then unable to replenish the nutrients at a rate fast enough to maintain maximum force for long. As a result, the maximum force the muscle is capable of producing is limited by the bottleneck in nutrient availability, and decreases exponentially.

Imagine a theoretical arm wrestling match with two perfectly matched opponents, each exactly as strong as each other. They both begin the match by exerting maximum force on each other's hands, but very soon, their arms get fatigued and the actual force being exerted on each other's hands drops off quickly. They are still exerting as much force as they can, but their muscles are burning energy faster than can be replenished, and their maximum force is decreasing exponentially. Eventually their arms are completely fatigued; they are basically just holding hands and applying what little force their muscles can muster, wondering when the other will give up.

Rohmert's law suggests that, for example, static gripping loads be not more than 15% of the load required for a squeeze-operated tool.

While Rohmert's law applies to *maximum* force, the inverse is true as well; the less force one is asked to exert, the longer one will be able to exert that force before their muscles become fatigued. If one is asked to exert zero force, they can theoretically hold the position indefinitely.

Rohmert's law has been found to be true across all humans. While everyone has a different initial maximum force they can apply, their maximum force will decrease according to the same exponential curve as everyone else.

Engineering Psychology

Engineering psychology is the science of human behavior and capability, applied to the design and operation of systems and technology. As an applied field of psychology and an interdisciplinary part of ergonomics, it aims to improve the relationships between people and machines by redesigning equipment, interactions, or the environment in which they take place. The work of an engineering psychologist is often described as making the relationship more "user-friendly."

History

Engineering psychology was created from within experimental psychology. Engineering psychology started during World War I (1914). The reason why this subject was developed during this time was because many of America's weapons were failing; bombs not falling in the right place to weapons attacking normal marine life. The fault was traced back to human errors. One of the first designs to be built to restrain human error was the use of psychoacoustics by S.S. Stevens and L.L. Beranek were two of the first American psychologists called upon to help change how people and machinery worked together. One of their first assignments was to try and reduce noise levels in military aircraft. The work was directed at improving intelligibility of military communication systems and appeared to have been very successful. However it was not until after August 1945 that levels of research in engineering psychology began to increase significantly. This occurred because the research that started in 1940 now began to show.

Lillian Gilbreth combined the talents of an engineer, psychologist and mother of twelve. Her appreciation of human factors made her successful in the implementation of time and motion studies and scientific management. She went on to pioneer ergonomics in the kitchen, inventing the pedal bin, for example.

In Britain, the two world wars generated much formal study of human factors which affected the efficiency of munitions output and warfare. In World War I, the Health of Munitions Workers Committee was created in 1915. This made recommendations based upon studies of the effects of overwork on efficiency which resulted in policies of providing breaks and limiting hours of work, including avoidance of work on Sunday. The Industrial Fatigue Research Board was created in 1918 to take this work forward. In WW2, researchers at Cambridge University such as Frederic Bartlett and Kenneth Craik started work on the operation of equipment in 1939 and this resulted in the creation of the Unit for Research in Applied Psychology in 1944.

Related Subjects

- Cognitive ergonomics & cognitive engineering - studies cognition in work settings, in order to optimize *human well-being and system performance.* It is a subset of the larger field of human factors and ergonomics.
- Applied psychology - The use of psychological principles to overcome problems in other domains. It has been argued that engineering psychology is separate from applied (cognitive) psychology because advances in cognitive psychology have infrequently informed engineering psychology research. Surprisingly, work in engineering psychology often seems to inform developments in cognitive psychology. For example, engineering psychology research has enabled cognitive psychologists to explain why GUIs seem easier to use than character-based computer interfaces (such as DOS).

Engineering Psychology, Ergonomics, & Human Factors

Although the comparability of these terms and many others have been a topic of debate, the differences of these fields can be seen in the applications of the respective fields.

Engineering psychology is concerned with the adaptation of the equipment and environment to people, based upon their psychological capacities and limitations with the objective of improving overall system performance, involving human and machine elements Engineering psychologists strive to match equipment requirements with the capabilities of human operators by changing the design of the equipment. An example of this matching was the redesign of the mailbags used by letter carriers. Engineering psychologists discovered that mailbag with a waist-support strap, and a double bag that requires the use of both shoulders, reduces muscle fatigue. Another example involves the cumulative trauma disorders grocery checkout workers suffered as the result of repetitive wrist movements using electronic scanners. Engineering psychologists found that the optimal checkout station design would allow for workers to easily use either hand to distribute the workload between both wrists.

The field of ergonomics is based on scientific studies of ordinary people in work situations and is applied to the design of processes and machines, to the layout of work places, to methods of work, and to the control of the physical environment, in order to achieve greater efficiency of both men and machines An example of an ergonomics study is the evaluation of the effects of screwdriver handle shape, surface material and workpiece orientation on torque performance, finger force distribution and muscle activity in a maximum screwdriving torque task. Another example of an ergonomics study is the effects of shoe traction and obstacle height on friction. Similarly, many topics in ergonomics deal with the actual science of matching man to equipment and encompasses narrower fields such as Engineering Psychology.

At one point in time, the term human factors was used in place of ergonomics in Europe. Human factors involve interdisciplinary scientific research and studies to seek to realize greater recognition and understanding of the worker's characteristics, needs, abilities, and limitations when the procedures and products of technology are being designed. This field utilizes knowledge from several fields such as mechanical engineering, psychology, and industrial engineering to design instruments.

Human factors is broader than engineering psychology, which is focused specifically on designing systems that accommodate the information-processing capabilities of the brain.

Although the work in the respective fields differ, there are some similarities between these. These fields share the same objectives which are to optimize the effectiveness and efficiency with which human activities are conducted as well as to improve the general quality of life through increased safety, reduced fatigue and stress, increased comfort, and satisfaction.

Importance of Engineering Psychologists

Engineering psychologists contribute to the design of a variety of products, including dental and surgical tools, cameras, toothbrushes and car-seats. They have been involved in the re-design of the mailbags used by letter carriers. More than 20% of letter carriers suffer from musculoskeletal injury such as lower back pain from carrying mailbags slung over their shoulders. A mailbag with a waist-support strap, and a double bag that requires the use of both shoulders, has been shown to reduce muscle fatigue.

Research by engineering psychologists has demonstrated that using cell-phones while driving degrades performance by increasing driver reaction time, particularly among older drivers, and can lead to higher accident risk among drivers of all ages. Research findings such as these have supported governmental regulation of cell-phone use.

Industrial and Organizational Psychology

Industrial and organizational psychology (I/O psychology), also known as occupational psychology, organizational psychology, and work and organizational psychology, is an applied discipline within psychology. I/O psychology is the science of human behaviour relating to work and applies psychological theories and principles to organizations and individuals in their places of work as well as the individual's work-life more generally. I/O psychologists are trained in the scientist–practitioner model. I/O psychologists contribute to an organization's success by improving the performance, motivation, job satisfaction, and occupational safety and health as well as the overall health and well-being of its employees. An I/O psychologist conducts research on employee behaviours and attitudes, and how these can be improved through hiring practices, training programs, feedback, and management systems.

I/O psychology is one of the 15 recognized specialties in professional psychology in the United States. It is represented by Division 14 of the American Psychological Association (APA), known formally as the Society for Industrial and Organizational Psychology (SIOP). In the United Kingdom, industrial and organizational psychologists are referred to as occupational psychologists. Occupational psychology in the UK is one of nine 'protected titles' within the profession "practitioner psychologist" regulated by the Health and Care Professions Council. In the UK, graduate programs in psychology, including occupational psychology, are accredited by the British Psychological Society. To become an occupational psychologist in the UK, a doctorate is required.

In Australia, the title organizational psychologist is protected by law, and regulated by the Australian Health Practitioner Regulation Agency (AHPRA). Organizational psychology is one of nine areas of specialist endorsement for psychology practice in Australia.

In Europe someone with a specialist EuroPsy Certificate in Work and Organisational Psychology is a fully qualified psychologist and an expert in the work psychology field. Industrial and organizational psychologists reaching the EuroPsy standard are recorded in the Register of European Psychologists and industrial and organizational psychology is one of the three main psychology specializations in Europe.

Historical Overview

The historical development of I/O psychology was paralleled in the US, the UK, Australia, Germany, the Netherlands, and eastern European countries such as Romania. The roots of I/O psychology trace back nearly to the beginning of psychology as a science, when Wilhelm Wundt founded one of the first psychological laboratories in 1876 in Leipzig, Germany. In the mid 1880s, Wundt trained two psychologists, Hugo Münsterberg and James McKeen Cattell, who had a major influence on the emergence of I/O psychology.

Instead of viewing performance differences as human "errors", Cattell was one of the first to recognize the importance of differences among individuals as a way of better understanding work behavior. Walter Dill Scott, who was a contemporary of Cattell, was elected President of the American Psychological Association (APA) in 1919, was arguably the most prominent I/O psychologist of his time. Scott, along with Walter Van Dyke Bingham, worked at the Carnegie Institute of Technology, developing methods for selecting and training sales personnel.

The "industrial" side of I/O psychology originated in research on individual differences, assessment, and the prediction of work performance. Industrial psychology crystallized during World War I, in response to the need to rapidly assign new troops to duty. Scott and Bingham volunteered to help with the testing and placement of more than a million army recruits. In 1917, together with other prominent psychologists, they adapted a well-known intelligence test the Stanford–Binet, which was designed for testing one individual at a time, to make it suitable for group testing. The new test was called the Army Alpha.

After the War, the growing industrial base in the US was a source of momentum for what was then called industrial psychology. Private industry set out to emulate the successful testing of army personnel. Mental ability testing soon became commonplace in the work setting.

Elton Mayo found that rest periods improved morale and reduced turnover in a Philadelphia textile factory. He later joined the ongoing Hawthorne studies, where he became interested in how workers' emotions and informal relationships affected productivity. The results of these studies ushered in the human relations movement.

World War II brought renewed interest in ability testing (to accurately place recruits in new technologically advanced military jobs), the introduction of the assessment center, and concern with morale and fatigue in war industry workers.

The industrial psychology division of the former American Association of Applied Psychology became a division within APA, becoming Division 14 of APA. It was initially called the Industrial and Business Psychology Division. In 1962, the name was changed to the Industrial Psychology Division. In 1973, it was renamed again, this time to the Division of Industrial and Organizational Psychology. In 1982, the unit become more independent of APA, and its name was changed again, this time to the Society for Industrial and Organizational Psychology.

The name change of the division from "industrial psychology" to "industrial and organizational psychology" reflected the shift in the work of industrial psychologists who had originally addressed work behavior from the individual perspective, examining performance and attitudes of individual workers. Their work became broader. Group behavior in the workplace became a worthy subject of study. The emphasis on "organizational" underlined the fact that when an individual joins an organization (e.g., the organization that hired him or her), he or she will be exposed to a common goal and a common set of operating procedures. In the 1970s in the UK, references to occupational psychology became more common than I/O psychology.

According to Bryan and Vinchur, "while organizational psychology increased in popularity through [the 1960s and 1970s], research and practice in the traditional areas of industrial psychology continued, primarily driven by employment legislation and case law". There was a focus on fairness and validity in selection efforts as well as in the job analyses that undergirded selection instruments. For example, i/o psychology showed increased interest in behaviorally anchored rating scales. What critics there were of i/o psychology accused the discipline of being responsive only to the concerns of managements.

From the 1980 to 2010s other changes in i/o psychology took place. Researchers increasingly adopted a multi-level approach, attempting to understand behavioral phenomena from both the level of the organization and the level of the individual worker. There was also an increased interest in the needs and expectations of employees as individuals. For example, an emphasis on organizational justice and the psychological contract took root, as well as the more traditional concerns of selection and training. Methodological innovations (e.g., meta-analyses, structural equation modeling) were adopted. With the passage of the American with Disabilities Act in 1990 and parallel legislation elsewhere in the world, i/o psychology saw an increased emphasis on "fairness in personnel decisions." Training research relied increasingly on advances in educational psychology and cognitive science.

Research Methods

As described above, I/O psychologists are trained in the scientist–practitioner model. I/O psychologists rely on a variety of methods to conduct organizational research. Study designs employed by I/O psychologists include surveys, experiments, quasi-experiments, and observational studies. I/O psychologists rely on diverse data sources including human judgments, historical databases, objective measures of work performance (e.g., sales volume), and questionnaires and surveys.

I/O researchers employ quantitative statistical methods. Quantitative methods used in I/O psychology include correlation, multiple regression, and analysis of variance. More advanced statistical methods employed in I/O research include logistic regression, structural equation modeling, and hierarchical linear modeling (HLM; also known as multilevel modeling). I/O research has also employed meta-analysis. I/O psychologists also employ psychometric methods including methods associated with classical test theory, generalizability theory, and item response theory (IRT).

I/O psychologists have also employed qualitative methods, which largely involve focus groups, interviews, and case studies. I/O research on organizational culture research has employed ethnographic techniques and participant observation. A qualitative technique associated with I/O psychology is Flanagan's Critical Incident Technique. I/O psychologists sometimes use quantitative and qualitative methods in concert. OHP researchers have also combined and coordinated quantitative and qualitative methods within a single study.

Topics

Job Analysis

Job analysis encompasses a number of different methods. It primarily involves the systematic collection of information about a job. A task-oriented job analysis involves an examination of the duties, tasks, and/or competencies required by the job being assessed. By contrast, a worker-oriented job analysis involves an examination of the knowledge, skills, abilities, and other characteristics (KSAOs) required to successfully perform the work. Information obtained from job analyses are used for many purposes, including the creation of job-relevant selection procedures, performance appraisals and the criteria they require, and the development of training programs.

Personnel Recruitment and Selection

I/O psychologists typically work with human resource specialists to design (a) recruitment processes and (b) personnel selection systems. Personnel recruitment is the process of identifying qualified candidates in the workforce and getting them to apply for jobs within an organization. Personnel recruitment processes include developing job announcements, placing ads, defining key qualifications for applicants, and screening out unqualified applicants.

Personnel selection is the systematic process of hiring and promoting personnel. Personnel selection systems employ evidence-based practices to determine the most qualified candidates. Personnel selection involves both the newly hired and individuals who can be promoted from within the organization. Common selection tools include ability tests (e.g., cognitive, physical, or psycho-motor), knowledge tests, personality tests, structured interviews, the systematic collection of biographical data, and work samples. I/O psychologists must evaluate evidence regarding the extent to which selection tools predict job performance.

Personnel selection procedures are usually validated, i.e., shown to be job relevant to personnel selection, using one or more of the following types of validity: content validity, construct validity, and/or criterion-related validity. I/O psychologists must adhere to professional standards in personnel selection efforts. SIOP (e.g., *Principles for validation and use of personnel selection procedures*) and APA together with the National Council on Measurement in Education (e.g., *Standards for educational and psychological testing* are sources of those standards. The Equal Employment Opportunity Commission's *Uniform guidelines* are also influential in guiding personnel selection decisions.

A meta-analysis of selection methods found that general mental ability was the best overall predictor of job performance and attainment in training.

Performance Appraisal/Management

Performance appraisal or performance evaluation is the process in which an individual's or a group's work behaviors and outcomes are assessed against managers' and others' expectations for the job. Performance appraisal is frequently used in promotion and compensation decisions, to help design and validate personnel selection procedures, and for performance management. Performance management is the process of providing performance feedback relative to expectations, and information relevant to improvement (e.g., coaching, mentoring). Performance management may also include documenting and tracking performance information for organizational evaluation purposes.

An I/O psychologist would typically use information from the job analysis to determine a job's performance dimensions, and then construct a rating scale to describe each level of performance for the job. Often, the I/O psychologist would be responsible for training organizational personnel how to use the performance appraisal instrument, including ways to minimize bias when using the rating scale, and how to provide effective performance feedback.

Individual Assessment and Psychometrics

Individual assessment involves the measurement of individual differences. I/O psychologists perform individual assessments in order to evaluate differences among candidates for employment as well as differences among employees. The constructs measured pertain to job performance. With candidates for employment, individual assessment is often part of the personnel selection process. These assessments can include written tests, aptitude tests, physical tests, psycho-motor tests, personality tests, integrity and reliability tests, work samples, simulations, and assessment centres.

Occupational Health and Well-being

I/O psychologists are concerned with occupational health and well-being. Early in the 20th century Arthur Kornhauser examined the impact on productivity of hiring mentally unstable workers. Kornhauser also examined the link between industrial working conditions and mental health as well as the spillover into a worker's personal life of having an unsatisfying job.

More recently, I/O researchers have found that staying vigorous during working hours is associated with better work-related behaviour and subjective well-being as well as more effective functioning in the family domain. Trait vigor and recovery experiences after work were related to vigor at work. Job satisfaction has also been found to be associated with life satisfaction, happiness, well-being and positive affect, and the absence of negative affect. Other research indicates that among older workers activities such as volunteering and participating in social clubs was related to a decrease in depressive symptoms over the next two years. Research on job changing indicates that mobility between, but not within, organizations is associated with burnout.

Workplace Bullying, Aggression and Violence

I/O psychologists are concerned with the related topics of workplace bullying, aggression, and violence. For example, I/O research found that exposure to workplace violence elicited ruminative thinking, and ruminative thinking, in turn, is associated with poor well-being. I/O research has found that interpersonal aggressive behaviours is associated with worse team performance.

Remuneration and Compensation

Compensation includes wages or salary, bonuses, pension/retirement contributions, and employee benefits that can be converted to cash or replace living expenses. I/O psychologists may be asked to conduct a job evaluation for the purpose of determining compensation levels and ranges. I/O psychologists may also serve as expert witnesses in pay discrimination cases, when disparities in pay for similar work are alleged by employees.

Training and Training Evaluation

Training involves the systematic teaching of skills, concepts, or attitudes that results in improved performance in another environment. Because many people hired for a job are not already versed in all the tasks the job requires, training may be needed to help the individual perform the job effectively. Evidence indicates that training is often effective, and that it succeeds in terms of higher net sales and gross profitability per employee.

Similar to performance management, an I/O psychologist would employ a job analysis in concert with the application of the principles of instructional design to create an effective training program. A training program is likely to include a summative evaluation at its conclusion in order to ensure that trainees have met the training objectives and can perform the target work tasks at an acceptable level. Training programs often include formative evaluations to assess the effect of the training as the training proceeds. Formative evaluations can be used to locate problems in training procedures and help I/O psychologists make corrective adjustments while training is ongoing.

The foundation for training programs is learning. Learning outcomes can be organized into three broad categories: cognitive, skill-based, and affective outcomes. Cognitive training is aimed at instilling declarative knowledge or the knowledge of rules, facts, and principles (e.g., police officer training covers laws and court procedures). Skill-based training aims to impart procedural knowledge (e.g., skills needed to use a special tool) or technical skills (e.g., understanding the workings of software program). Affective training concerns teaching individuals to develop specific attitudes or beliefs that predispose trainees to behave a certain way (e.g., show commitment to the organization, appreciate diversity).

A needs assessment, an analysis of corporate and individual goals, is often undertaken prior to the development of a training program. In addition, a careful needs analysis is required in order to develop a systematic understanding of where training is needed, what should be taught, and who will be trained. A training needs analysis typically involves a three-step process that includes organizational analysis, task analysis and person analysis.

An organizational analysis is an examination of organizational goals and resources as well as the organizational environment. The results of an organizational analysis help to determine where training should be directed. The analysis identifies the training needs of different departments or subunits. It systematically assesses manager, peer, and technological support for transfer of training. An organizational analysis also takes into account the climate of the organization and its subunits. For example, if a climate for safety is emphasized throughout the organization or in subunits of the organization (e.g., production), then training needs will likely reflect an emphasis on safety. A task analysis uses the results of a job analysis to determine what is needed for successful job performance, contributing to training content. With organizations increasingly trying to identify "core competencies" that are required for all jobs, task analysis can also include an assessment of competencies. A person analysis identifies which individuals within an organization should receive training and what kind of instruction they need. Employee needs can be assessed using a variety of methods that identify weaknesses that training can address.

Motivation in the Workplace

Work motivation reflects the energy an individual applies "to initiate work-related behavior, and to determine its form, direction, intensity, and duration" Understanding what motivates an organization's employees is central to I/O psychology. Motivation is generally thought of as a theoretical construct that fuels behavior. An incentive is an anticipated reward that is thought to incline a person to behave a certain way. Motivation varies among individuals. Studying its influence on behavior, it must be examined together with ability and environmental influences. Because of motivation's role in influencing workplace behavior and performance, many organizations structure the work environment to encourage productive behaviors and discourage unproductive behaviors.

Motivation involves three psychological processes: arousal, direction, and intensity. Arousal is what initiates action. It is often fueled by a person's need or desire for something that is missing from his or her life, either totally or partially. Direction refers to the path employees take in accomplishing the goals they set for themselves. Intensity is the amount of energy employees put into goal-directed work performance. The level of intensity often reflects the importance and difficulty of the goal. These psychological processes involve four factors. First, motivation serves to direct attention, focusing on particular issues, people, tasks, etc. Second, it serves to stimulate effort. Third, motivation influences persistence. Finally, motivation influences the choice and application of task-related strategies.

Occupational Stress

I/O psychologists are involved in the research and the practice of occupational stress and design of individual and organizational interventions to manage and reduce the stress levels and increase productivity, performance, health and wellbeing. Occupational stress can have implications for organizational performance because of the emotions job stress evokes. For example, a job stressor such as conflict with a supervisor can precipitate anger that in turn motivates counterproductive workplace behaviors. I/O research has examined the association between work stressors and aggression, theft, substance abuse, and depressive symptoms. A number of models have been developed to explain the job stress process, including the person-environment fit model and the demand-control model. Those models became a cornerstone of the emergence, in the late 1980s and early 1990s, of a new discipline relevant to research on occupational stress; the discipline, occupational health psychology, is an offshoot of i/o psychology, health psychology, and occupational medicine.

Research has also examined occupational stress in specific occupations, including police, general practitioners, and dentists. Another concern has been the relation of occupational stress to family life. Other research has examined gender differences in leadership style and job stress and strain in the context of male- and female-dominated industries, and unemployment-related distress. I/O psychology is also concerned with the relation of occupational stress to career advancement.

Occupational Safety

Accidents and safety in the workplace have become areas of interest to I/O psychology. Examples of psychosocial injury hazards of interest to I/O psychology include fatigue, workplace violence, workplace bullying, and working night shifts. I/O researchers conduct "stress audits" that can help organizations remain compliant with various occupational safety regulations. Psychosocial hazards can affect musculoskeletal disorders. A psychosocial factor related to accident risk is safety climate, which refers to employees' perceptions of the extent to which their work organization prioritizes safety. By contrast, psychosocial safety climate refers to management's "policies, practices, and procedures" aimed at protecting workers' psychological health. Research on safety leadership is also relevant to I/O psychology. Research suggests that safety-oriented transformational leadership is associated with a positive safety climate and safe worker practices.

Organizational Culture

Organizational culture has been described as a set of assumptions shared by individuals in an organization; the assumptions influence the interpretation and actions that define appropriate behavior for various situations. Organizational culture has been shown to affect important organizational outcomes such as performance, attraction, recruitment, retention, employee satisfaction, and employee well-being. There are three levels of organizational culture: artifacts, shared values, and basic beliefs and assumptions. Artifacts comprise the physical components of the organization that relay cultural meaning. Shared values are individuals' preferences regarding certain aspects of the organization's culture (e.g., loyalty, customer service). Basic beliefs and assumptions include individuals' impressions about the trustworthiness and supportiveness of an organization, and are often deeply ingrained within the organization's culture.

In addition to an overall culture, organizations also have subcultures. Examples of subcultures include corporate culture, departmental culture, local culture, and issue-related culture. While there is no single "type" of organizational culture, some researchers have developed models to describe different organizational cultures.

Group Behavior

Group behavior involves the interactions among individuals in a collective. The individuals' opinions, attitudes, and adaptations affect group behavior and group behavior, in turn, affects those opinions, etc. The interactions are thought to fulfill some need satisfaction in an individual who is part of the collective. A specific area of I/O research in group behavior is the team dynamics and team effectiveness.

Team Effectiveness

Organizations often organize teams because teams can accomplish a much greater amount of work in a short period of time than an individual can accomplish. I/O research has examined the harm workplace aggression does to team performance.

Team Composition

The selection of individuals to be assigned to specific teams bears on the resulting effectiveness of those teams. Aspects of team composition that should be considered during the team selection process include team members' knowledge, skills, and abilities (KSAs) as well their personalities and attitudes. To achieve high-quality results, teams built with members having higher skill levels are more likely to be effective than teams built around members having lesser skills; teams that include a members with a diversity of skills are also likely to show improved team performance. Additionally, higher levels of cognitive ability of team members has been shown to consistently correlate to increased work group effectiveness. Team members' personalities and attitudes have also been studied. For example, the personality factors agreeableness, conscientiousness, extraversion, and emotional stability are related to better team performance.

Task Design

A fundamental question in team task design is whether or not a task is even appropriate for a team. Those tasks that require predominantly independent work are best left to individuals, and team tasks should include those tasks that consist primarily of interdependent work. When a given task is appropriate for a team, task design can play a key role in team effectiveness.

Job characteristic theory identifies core job dimensions that affect motivation, satisfaction, performance, etc. These dimensions include skill variety, task identity, task significance, autonomy and feedback. The dimensions map well to the team environment. Individual contributors who perform team tasks that are challenging, interesting, and engaging are more likely to be motivated to exert greater effort and perform better than team members who are working on tasks that lack those characteristics.

Organizational Resources

Organizational support systems affect the team effectiveness and provide resources for teams operating in the multi-team environment. During the chartering of new teams, organizational enabling resources are first identified. Examples of enabling resources include facilities, equipment, information, training, and leadership. Team-specific resources (e.g., budgetary resources, human resources) are typically made available. Team-specific human resources represent the individual contributors who are selected to be team members. Intra-team processes (e.g., task design, task assignment) involve these team-specific resources.

Teams also function in dynamic multi-team environments. Teams often must respond to shifting organizational contingencies. Contingencies affecting teams include constraints arising from conditions in which organizational resources are not exclusively earmarked for certain teams. When resources are scarce, they must be shared by multiple teams.

Team Rewards

Organizational reward systems drive the strengthening and enhancing of individual team member efforts; such efforts contribute towards reaching team goals. In other words, rewards that are given to individual team members should be contingent upon the performance of the entire team.

Several design elements are needed to enable organizational reward systems to operate successfully. First, for a collective assessment to be appropriate for individual team members, the group's tasks must be highly interdependent. If this is not the case, individual assessment is more appropriate than team assessment. Second, individual-level reward systems and team-level reward systems must be compatible. For example, it would be unfair to reward the entire team for a job well done if only one team member did most of the work. That team member would most likely view teams and teamwork negatively, and would not want to work on a team in the future. Third, an organizational culture must be created such that it supports and rewards employees who believe in the value of teamwork and who maintain a positive attitude towards team-based rewards.

Team Goals

Goals potentially motivate team members when goals contain three elements: difficulty, acceptance, and specificity. Under difficult goal conditions, teams with more committed members tend to outperform teams with less committed members. When team members commit to team goals, team effectiveness is a function of how supportive members are with each other. The goals of individual team members and team goals interact. Team and individual goals must be coordinated. Individual goals must be consistent with team goals in order for a team to be effective.

Job Satisfaction and Commitment

Job satisfaction is often thought to reflect the extent to which a worker likes his or her job, or individual aspects or facets of jobs. It is one of the most heavily researched topics in I/O psychology. Job satisfaction has theoretical and practical utility for the field. It has been linked to important job outcomes including attitudinal variables (e.g., job involvement, organizational commitment), absenteeism, turnover intentions, actual turnover, job performance, and tension. A meta-analyses found job satisfaction to be related to life satisfaction, happiness, positive affect, and the absence of negative affect.

Productive Behavior

Productive behavior is defined as employee behavior that contributes positively to the goals and objectives of an organization. When an employee begins a new job, there is a transition period during which he or she may not contribute significantly. To assist with this transition an employee typically requires job-related training. In financial terms, productive behavior represents the point at which an organization begins to achieve some return on the investment it has made in a new employee. I/O psychologists are ordinarily more focused on productive behavior than job or task performance, including in-role *and* extra-role performance. In-role performance tells managers how well an employee performs the required aspects of the job; extra-role performance includes behaviors not necessarily required by job but nonetheless contribute to organizational effectiveness. By taking both in-role and extra-role performance into account, an I/O psychologist is able to assess employees' effectiveness (how well they do what they were hired to do), efficiency (outputs to relative inputs), and productivity (how much they help the organization reach its goals). Three forms of productive behavior that I/O psychologists often evaluate include job performance, organizational citizenship behavior, and innovation.

Job Performance

Job performance represents behaviors employees engage in while at work which contribute to organizational goals. These behaviors are formally evaluated by an organization as part of an employee's responsibilities. In order to understand and ultimately predict job performance, it is important to be precise when defining the term. Job performance is about behaviors that are within the control of the employee and not about results (effectiveness), the costs involved in achieving results (productivity), the results that can be achieved in a period of time (efficiency), or the value an organization places on a given level of performance, effectiveness, productivity or efficiency (utility).

To model job performance, researchers have attempted to define a set of dimensions that are common to all jobs. Using a common set of dimensions provides a consistent basis for assessing performance and enables the comparison of performance across jobs. Performance is commonly broken into two major categories: in-role (technical aspects of a job) and extra-role (non-technical abilities such as communication skills and being a good team member). While this distinction in behavior has been challenged it is commonly made by both employees and management. A model of performance by Campbell breaks performance into in-role and extra-role categories. Campbell labeled job-specific task proficiency and non-job-specific task proficiency as in-role dimensions, while written and oral communication, demonstrating effort, maintaining personal discipline, facilitating peer and team performance, supervision and leadership and management and administration are labeled as extra-role dimensions. Murphy's model of job performance also broke job performance into in-role and extra-role categories. However, task-orientated behaviors composed the in-role category and the extra-role category included interpersonally-oriented behaviors, down-time behaviors and destructive and hazardous behaviors. However, it has been challenged as to whether the measurement of job performance is usually done through pencil/paper tests, job skills tests, on-site hands-on tests, off-site hands-on tests, high-fidelity simulations, symbolic simulations, task ratings and global ratings. These various tools are often used to evaluate performance on specific tasks and overall job performance. Van Dyne and LePine developed a measurement model in which overall job performance was evaluated using Campbell's in-role and extra-role categories. Here, in-role performance was reflected through how well "employees met their performance expectations and performed well at the tasks that made up the employees' job." Dimensions regarding how well the employee assists others with their work for the benefit of the group, if the employee voices new ideas for projects or changes to procedure and whether the employee attends functions that help the group composed the extra-role category.

To assess job performance, reliable and valid measures must be established. While there are many sources of error with performance ratings, error can be reduced through rater training and through the use of behaviorally-anchored rating scales. Such scales can be used to clearly define the behaviors that constitute poor, average, and superior performance. Additional factors that complicate the measurement of job performance include the instability of job performance over time due to forces such as changing performance criteria, the structure of the job itself and the restriction of variation in individual performance by organizational forces. These factors include errors in job measurement techniques, acceptance and the justification of poor performance and lack of importance of individual performance.

The determinants of job performance consist of factors having to do with the individual worker as well as environmental factors in the workplace. According to Campbell's Model of The Determinants of Job Performance, job performance is a result of the interaction between declarative knowledge (knowledge of facts or things), procedural knowledge (knowledge of what needs to be done and how to do it), and motivation (reflective of an employee's choices regarding whether to expend effort, the level of effort to expend, and whether to persist with the level of effort chosen). The interplay between these factors show that an employee may, for example, have a low level of declarative knowledge, but may still have a high level of performance if the employee has high levels of procedural knowledge and motivation.

Regardless of the job, three determinants stand out as predictors of performance: (1) general mental ability (especially for jobs higher in complexity); (2) job experience (although there is a law of diminishing returns); and (3) the personality trait of conscientiousness (people who are dependable and achievement-oriented, who plan well). These determinants appear to influence performance largely through the acquisition and usage of job knowledge and the motivation to do well. Further, an expanding area of research in job performance determinants includes emotional intelligence.

Organizational Citizenship Behavior

Organizational citizenship behaviors (OCBs) are another form of workplace behavior that I/O psychologists are involved with. OCBs tend to be beneficial to both the organization and other workers. Dennis Organ (1988) defines OCBs as "individual behavior that is discretionary, not directly or explicitly recognized by the formal reward system, and that in the aggregate promotes the effective functioning of the organization." Behaviors that qualify as OCBs can fall into one of the following five categories: altruism, courtesy, sportsmanship, conscientiousness, and civic virtue. OCBs have also been categorized in other ways too, for example, by their intended targets (individuals, supervisors, and the organization as a whole. Other alternative ways of categorizing OCBs include "compulsory OCBs," which are engaged in owing to coercive persuasion or peer pressure rather than out of good will. The extent to which OCBs are voluntary has been the subject of some debate.

Other research suggests that some employees perform OCBs to influence how they are viewed within the organization. While these behaviors are not formally part of the job description, performing them can influence performance appraisals. Researchers have advanced the view that employees engage in OCBs as a form of "impression management," a term coined by Erving Goffman. Goffman defined impression management as "the way in which the individual ... presents himself and his activity to others, the ways in which he guides and controls the impression they form of him, and the kinds of things he may and may not do while sustaining his performance before them. Some researchers have hypothesized that OCBs are not performed out of good will, positive affect, etc., but instead as a way of being noticed by others, including supervisors.

Innovation

Industrial and organizational psychologists consider innovation, more often than not, a variable of less importance and often a counter-productive one to include in conducting job performance appraisals when irrelevant to the major job functions for which a given job exists. Nonetheless, I/O psychologists see the value of that variable where its consideration would, were its reliability and validity questioned, achieve a statistically significant probability that its results are not due to chance, and that it can be replicated reliably with a statistically significant ratio of reliability, and that were a court to raise a question on its reliability and validity testing, the I/O psychologist behind its use would be able to defend it before a court of justice with the belief that it will stand before such a court as reliable, and valid.

Four qualities are generally linked to creative and innovative behaviour by individuals:

- Task-relevant skills (general mental ability and job specific knowledge). Task specific and subject specific knowledge is most often gained through higher education; however, it may also be gained by mentoring and experience in a given field.
- Creativity-relevant skills (ability to concentrate on a problem for long periods of time, to abandon unproductive searches, and to temporarily put aside stubborn problems). The ability to put aside stubborn problems is referred to by Jex & Britt as productive forgetting. Creativity-relevant skills also require the individual contributor to evaluate a problem from multiple vantage points. One must be able to take on the perspective of various users. For example, an Operation Manager analyzing a reporting issue and developing an innovative solution would consider the perspective of a sales person, assistant, finance, compensation, and compliance officer.
- Task motivation (internal desire to perform task and level of enjoyment).

At the organizational level, a study by Damanpour identified four specific characteristics that may predict innovation:

1. A population with high levels of technical knowledge
2. The organization's level of specialization

3. The level an organization communicates externally
4. Functional Differentiation.

Counterproductive Work Behavior

Counterproductive work behavior (CWB) can be defined as employee behavior that goes against the goals of an organization. These behaviors can be intentional or unintentional and result from a wide range of underlying causes and motivations. Some CWBs have instrumental motivations (e.g., theft). It has been proposed that a person-by-environment interaction can be utilized to explain a variety of counterproductive behaviors (Fox and Spector, 1999). For instance, an employee who sabotages another employee's work may do so because of lax supervision (environment) and underlying psychopathology (person) that work in concert to result in the counterproductive behavior. There is evidence that an emotional response (e.g., anger) to job stress (e.g., unfair treatment) can motivate CWBs.

The forms of counterproductive behavior with the most empirical examination are ineffective job performance, absenteeism, job turnover, and accidents. Less common but potentially more detrimental forms of counterproductive behavior have also been investigated including violence and sexual harassment.

Leadership

In I/O psychology, leadership can be defined as a process of influencing others to agree on a shared purpose, and to work towards shared objectives. A distinction should be made between leadership and management. Managers process administrative tasks and organize work environments. Although leaders may be required to undertake managerial duties as well, leaders typically focus on inspiring followers and creating a shared organizational culture and values. Managers deal with complexity, while leaders deal with initiating and adapting to change. Managers undertake the tasks of planning, budgeting, organizing, staffing, controlling and problem solving. In contrast, leaders undertake the tasks of setting a direction or vision, aligning people to shared goals, communicating, and motivating.

Approaches to studying leadership in I/O psychology can be broadly classified into three categories: Leader-focused approaches, contingency-focused approaches, and follower-focused approaches.

Leader-focused Approaches

Leader-focused approaches look to organizational leaders to determine the characteristics of effective leadership. According to the trait approach, more effective leaders possess certain traits that less effective leaders lack. More recently, this approach is being used to predict leader emergence. The following traits have been identified as those that predict leader emergence when there is no formal leader: high intelligence, high needs for dominance, high self-motivation, and socially perceptive. Another leader-focused approached is the behavioral approach which focuses on the behaviors that distinguish effective from ineffective leaders. There are two categories of leadership behaviors: (1) consideration; and (2) initiating structure. Behaviors associated with the category of consideration include showing subordinates they are valued and that the leader cares about them. An example of a consideration behavior is showing compassion when problems arise in or out of the office. Behaviors associated with the category of initiating structure include facilitating the task performance of groups. One example of an initiating structure behavior is meeting one-on-one with subordinates to explain expectations and goals. The final leader-focused approach is power and influence. To be most effective a leader should be able to influence others to behave in ways that are in line with the organization's mission and goals. How influential a leader can be depends on their social power or their potential to influence their subordinates. There are six bases of power: coercive power, reward power, legitimate power, expert power, referent power, and informational power. A leader can use several different tactics to influence others within an organization. These common tactics include: rational persuasion, inspirational appeal, consultation, ingratiation, exchange, personal appeal, coalition, legitimating, and pressure.

Contingency-focused Approaches

Of the 3 approaches to leadership, contingency-focused approaches have been the most prevalent over the past 30 years. Contingency-focused theories base a leader's effectiveness on their ability to assess a situation and adapt their behavior accordingly. These theories assume that an effective leader can accurately "read" a situation and skillfully employ a leadership style that meets the needs of the individuals involved and the task at hand. A brief introduction to the most prominent contingency-focused theories will follow.

Fiedler's Contingency Theory holds that a leader's effectiveness depends on the interaction between their characteristics and the characteristics of the situation. Path–Goal Theory asserts that the role of the leader is to help his or her subordinates achieve their goals. To effectively do this, leaders must skillfully select from four different leadership styles to meet the situational factors. The situational factors are a product of the characteristics of subordinates and the characteristics of the environment. The Leader-Member Exchange (LMX) Model focuses on how leader–subordinate relationships develop. Generally speaking, when a subordinate performs well or when there are positive exchanges between a leader and a subordinate, their relationship is strengthened, performance and job satisfaction are enhanced, and the subordinate will feel more commitment to the leader and the organization as a whole. Vroom-Yetton-Jago Model focuses on decision making with respect to a *feasibility set* which is composed of the situational attributes.

In addition to the contingency-focused approaches mentioned, there has been a high degree of interest paid to three novel approaches that have recently emerged. The first is transformational leadership, which posits that there are certain leadership traits that inspire subordinates to perform beyond their capabilities. The second is transactional leadership, which is most concerned with keeping subordinates in-line with deadlines and organizational policy. This type of leader fills more of a managerial role and lacks qualities necessary to inspire subordinates and induce meaningful change. And the third is authentic leadership which is centered around empathy and a leader's values or character. If the leader understands their followers, they can inspire subordinates by cultivating a personal connection and leading them to share in the vision and goals of the team. Although there has been a limited amount of research conducted on these theories, they are sure to receive continued attention as the field of I/O psychology matures.

Follower-focused Approaches

Follower-focused approaches look at the processes by which leaders motivate followers, and lead teams to achieve shared goals. Understandably, the area of leadership motivation draws heavily from the abundant research literature in the domain of motivation in I/O psychology. Because leaders are held responsible for their followers' ability to achieve the organization's goals, their ability to motivate their followers is a critical factor of leadership effectiveness. Similarly, the area of team leadership draws heavily from the research in teams and team effectiveness in I/O psychology. Because organizational employees are frequently structured in the form of teams, leaders need to be aware of the potential benefits and pitfalls of working in teams, how teams develop, how to satisfy team members' needs, and ultimately how to bring about team effectiveness and performance.

An emerging area of I/O research in the area of team leadership is in leading virtual teams, where people in the team are geographically-distributed across various distances and sometimes even countries. While technological advances have enabled the leadership process to take place in such virtual contexts, they present new challenges for leaders as well, such as the need to use technology to build relationships with followers, and influencing followers when faced with limited (or no) face-to-face interaction.

Organizational Development

I/O psychologists are also concerned with organizational change. This effort, called organizational development (OD). Tools used to advance organization development include the survey feedback technique. The technique involves the periodic assessment (with surveys) of employee attitudes and feelings. The results are conveyed to organizational stakeholders, who may want to take the organization in a particular direction. Another tool is the team building technique. Because many if not most tasks within the organization are completed by small groups and/or teams, team building is important to organizational success. In order to enhance a team's morale and problem-solving skills, I/O psychologists help the groups to build their self-confidence, group cohesiveness, and working effectiveness.

Relation to Organizational Behavior

The I/O psychology and organizational behavior have manifested some overlap. The overlap has led to some confusion regarding how the two disciplines differ.

Training

The minimum requirement for working as an I/O psychologist is a master's degree. Normally, this degree requires about 2–3 years to complete. Of all the degrees granted in I/O psychology each year, approximately two thirds are at the master's level.

A comprehensive list of US and Canadian master's and doctoral programs can be found at the web site of the Society for Industrial and Organizational Psychology (SIOP). Admission into I/O psychology PhD programs is highly competitive given that many programs accept a small number of applicants every year.

There are graduate degree programs in I/O psychology outside of the US and Canada. The SIOP web site also provides a comprehensive list of I/O programs in many other countries.

Competencies

There are many different sets of competencies for different specializations within I/O psychology and I/O psychologists are versatile behavioral scientists. For example, an I/O psychologist specializing in selection and recruiting should have expertise in finding the best talent for the organization and getting everyone on board while he or she might not need to know much about executive coaching. Some I/O psychologists specialize in specific areas of consulting whereas others tend to generalize their areas of expertise. There are basic skills and knowledge an individual needs in order to be an effective I/O psychologist, including include being an independent learner, interpersonal skills (e.g., listening skills), and general consultation skills (e.g., skills and knowledge in the problem area).

Job Outlook

According to the United States Department of Labor's Bureau of Labor Statistics, I/O psychology is the fastest growing occupation in the United States, based on projections between 2012 and 2022. In a 2006 salary survey, the median salary for a PhD in I/O psychology was $98,000; for a master's level I/O psychologist was $72,000. The highest paid PhD I/O psychologists in private industry worked in pharmaceuticals and averaged approximately $151,000 per year; the median salary for self-employed consultants was $150,000; those employed in retail, energy, and manufacturing followed closely behind, averaging approximately $133,000. The lowest earners were found in state and local government positions, averaging approximately $77,000. In 2005, I/O psychologists whose primary responsibility is teaching at private and public colleges and universities often earn additional income from consulting with government and industry.

Ethics

An I/O psychologist, whether an academic, a consultant, or an employee, must maintain high ethical standards. The APA's ethical principles apply to I/O psychologists. For example, ethically, the I/O psychologist should only accept projects for which he or she is qualified. With more organizations becoming global, it is important that when an I/O psychologist works outside her or his home country, the psychologist is aware of rules, regulations, and cultures of the organizations and countries in which the psychologist works, while adhering to the ethical standards set at home.

Workplace Aggression

Workplace aggression is a specific type of aggression which occurs in the workplace. Workplace aggression can include a wide range of behaviors, ranging from verbal acts (e.g., insulting someone or spreading rumors) to physical attacks (e.g., punching or slapping).

Definition

Aggression, in general, is any behavior an individual carries out with the intent to harm another person or group of people. The aggressor must believe that their behavior is harmful to their target, and that the target is motivated to avoid this behavior. A defining feature of aggression is the intent or motivation to harm. For a behavior to be considered an aggressive act, the individual committing the behavior must intend harm. In other words, if they inflict harm on another without that specific intent, it is not considered aggression.

Aggression can occur in a variety of situations. One important domain to understand aggression is in the workplace. Workplace aggression is considered a specific type of counterproductive work behavior (CWB) and is defined as "any act of aggression, physical assault, threatening or coercive behavior that causes physical or emotional harm in a work setting."

Some researchers specify that workplace aggression only includes efforts to harm coworkers, former coworkers, current employers, or past employers. Others include in workplace aggression any behaviors intended to harm another person that are enacted in a workplace.

Classification

To delineate the range of behaviors that can be considered aggressive workplace behaviors, researchers have developed schemes of classification for workplace aggression. Neuman and Baron (1998) offer these three dimensions that encompass the range of workplace aggression:

1. Expressions of hostility – behaviors that are primarily verbal or symbolic in nature
2. Obstructionism – behaviors intended to hinder an employee from performing their job or the organization from accomplishing its objectives
3. Overt aggression – violent acts

In an attempt to further break down the wide range of aggressive workplace behaviors, Baron and Neuman (1996) also classify workplace aggression based on these three dichotomies:

1. Verbal–physical
2. Direct–indirect
3. Active–passive

Aggressive acts can take any possible combination of these three dichotomies. For example, failing to deny false rumors about a coworker would be classified as verbal–passive–indirect. Purposely avoiding the presence of a coworker you know is searching for your assistance could be considered physical–passive–direct.

Other researchers offer a classification system based on the aggressor's relationship to the victim.

1. Criminal intent (Type I) – this type of aggression occurs when the aggressor has no relationship to the victim or organization.
2. Customer/client (Type II) – the aggressor has a relationship with the organization and aggresses while they are being served as a customer.
3. Worker on worker (Type III) – both the aggressor and the victim are employees in the same organization. Often, the aggressor is a supervisor, and the victim is a subordinate.
4. Personal relationship (Type IV) – the aggressor has a relationship with an employee at an organization, but not the organization itself. This category includes victims who are assaulted by a domestic partner while at work.

Covert Nature

In the workplace much of the aggressive behavior enacted on targets are considered covert in nature. According to Bjorkqvist, Osterman, and Hjelt-Back, covert behaviors are those behaviors that are designed to disguise the aggressive behavior or aggressive intentions from the target. Overt aggression, on the other hand, includes behaviors that do not hide the aggressive intent and are open in their intentions. Typically, covert aggression is verbal, indirect, and passive in nature, while overt aggression reflects the physical, direct, and active side of the dichotomies.

Workplace aggression often takes the form of covert behaviors. This can be attributed to what Bjorkqvist, Osterman, and Lagerspetz call the effect/danger ratio. This term refers to the aggressors' subjective evaluation of the relative effects and danger of committing an aggressive act. For an aggressor, it is ideal to have a larger effect/danger ratio. In other words, aggressors want an act to have a large effect with relatively low risk of danger to themselves.

Individuals in the workplace are subjected to prolonged exposure to each other. This prolonged exposure means the victims of the aggressors' actions likely have more time to retaliate, thus increasing the danger aspect of the ratio. Also, workplaces are often communal in nature. That is, people often work in groups and are surrounded by others. The presence of others acts as a sort of built in audience that could "punish" the aggressor for harming a victim. It is for these reasons that individuals often choose covert forms of aggression.

Predictors (Antecedents)

Predictors of workplace aggression can occur at both the organizational level and the individual level. Organizational factors examined here include organizational justice, supervision and surveillance, changes in the work environment, and specific job characteristics. At the individual level, gender, age, and alcohol consumption are examined here. While this is not a comprehensive listing of predictors, it does cover the majority of workplace aggression predictors addressed in the empirical literature.

Organizational (in) Justice

Perceived interpersonal justice, the degree to which people feel they are treated with fairness and respect, is negatively related to both psychological and physical aggression against supervisors. Inness, Barling, and Turner found similar results; perceived interpersonal injustice was related to workplace aggression in participants' primary and secondary jobs.

Moreover, perceived procedural justice, the extent to which formal organizational procedures are assumed fair, is related to workplace aggression against supervisors. Greenberg and Barling found that the greater the perceptions of procedural justice, the less workplace aggression was reported.

Termination and Job Security

The most extreme forms of workplace aggression may result from personnel decisions, such as individual termination and mass layoffs. In 2009 a man killed one and wounded five others at his former place of employment two years after he was let go from the company due to poor performance. A similar event occurred in 2012 when a man shot and killed four employees and then himself after losing his job earlier that day.

Downsizing is a tactic used by organizations where there is a slow-down in business in order to remain profitable or minimize losses. This tactic is most commonly observed during widespread economic hardships, such as the Great Recession of 2008.

Perceived job insecurity, or feelings of impending termination, has been found to be a predictor of workplace aggression.

Supervision and Surveillance

Workplace surveillance (employee monitoring) is positively related to workplace aggression against supervisors, such that the greater the number of employee surveillance methods used, the greater the amount of workplace aggression. Furthermore, supervisory control over work performance has also been shown positively related to workplace aggression against supervisors. This type of behavior has been observed both adults and teenagers.

Workplace Changes

Baron and Neuman found that certain changes in the work environment can lead to increased aggression that they attribute to heightened anxiety and stress. Specifically, pay cuts or freezes, changes in management, increased monitoring systems (e.g., increased computer monitoring), increased diversity, and the increased use of part-time employees all were related to higher levels of workplace aggression.

Job-specific Characteristics

Other antecedents of workplace aggression found in the literature are specific job characteristics. LeBlanc and Kelloway found that certain job features, such as handling guns or collecting valuable items, were significantly more related to workplace aggression.

Time Spent at Work

Harvey and Keashly found that length of time at work was able to predict workplace aggression such that the longer hours a person worked, the more likely they were to report aggression. The authors attributed this finding to two possible reasons. First, the more hours worked, the greater statistical probability of being victimized. Second, longer hours worked could contribute to fatigue and frustration. This in turn may increase the likelihood of aggressive actions towards coworkers.

Gender

In some studies, gender has been shown a significant predictor of workplace aggression. For example, being male is significantly related to reports of aggression against supervisors. Furthermore, males are more likely to commit aggressive acts in the presence of other men. This can be attributed to societal cultures that dictate "codes of honor." Females, on the other hand, are no more likely to act aggressively in either the presence of females or males.

Age

Age is significantly related to aggression. In their study of age and job performance, Ng and Feldman found that older workers (age 40 or older) engaged in less workplace aggression than younger workers.

Alcohol Consumption

The frequency and amount of alcohol typically consumed by a person predicts aggressive behavior. Those who consume more alcohol more frequently are more likely to aggress against a coworker. The Hebei tractor rampage began as workplace aggression following alcohol consumption.

Cyber-aggression

Cyber-aggression or cyber-harassment:

Takes the form of obscene or hate e-mail/text messages that threaten or frighten, or e-mails/text messages that contain offensive content, such as sexist or racist material. What is unique about this type of workplace harassment, compared to more traditional forms of harassment, is that this material can be sent by people in addition to work colleagues, by other individuals outside the workplace (either known or not known to the person) or even in the form of spam.

— Whitty & Carr,

What many do not realize that the phenomenon of cyber-bullying often associated with teenage culture has spread to the workplace in a variety of ways. While this trend is seemingly silent and slow growing, its effects are considered equally hurtful as any form of harassment.

Often, cyber-aggression is the result of individuals in a workplace being offended/upset/or feeling threatened by organizational problems. They then resort to virtual communication as a form of retaliation. These actions are referred to as *flaming* by Whitty & Carr, or essentially when an individual online writes with hostility towards a particular person or group of people.

Instant Messaging

Instant messaging has become both a help and a hindrance in organizations. The ease of use with instant messaging, is partially to blame, "Employees can see who else is available, and if it's someone they want to talk to, they're able to connect in real time". While this has become an extremely useful tool in workplace communication, instant messengers such at AIM or MSN Messenger are not easily regulated from a managerial aspect, which leads to employees being able to have private conversations on a public platform. These conversations can foster aggressive talk and lead to potentially hurtful information being spread among an organization. Some argue that instant messages are beneficial to the work process because it can easily resolve problems without having to distract the person via phone and you don't have to wait for an email response.

Email

This is one of the most prevalent tools used in cyber-aggression because of its prevalence in workplace communications. Often upset workers send loaded messages and attach the email to a large group of co-workers that are not involved in the issue to bring attention to it. An article from the Travel Trade Gazette give some advice to avoid being aggressive in emails.

- Always give a clear subject
- State exactly what you need in a simple manner
- Avoid terms like *ASAP*
- Only use reply all when it refers to the whole group
- Using all upper case is electronic SHOUTING!
- Don't use texting lexicon
- Never send an email when you are upset

Social Networking

This is one of the fastest growing ways that workers can lash out against each other. The opportunity is high for individuals to be aggressive in a highly public and open forum. Many choose to speak out at their co-workers or superiors because it is a way for them to vent their feelings while not having to say these things face to face.

Outcomes

Like the array of behaviors considered workplace aggression, the consequences of workplace aggression are also extensive. For example, Ng and Feldman suggest that "acts of workplace aggression can cause bodily harm to employees, pose physical danger for customers, create public relations crises, and harm the business reputation of the firm as a whole." The outcomes of workplace aggression addressed here include the health and well-being of targeted employees and job performance. Gender differences in outcomes are also addressed.

Severity of the repercussions may be influenced by the position of the aggressor. Hershcovis and Barling found that "...supervisor aggression has the strongest adverse effects across attitudinal and behavioral outcomes", followed by co-worker aggression and outsider aggression.

Health and Well-being

Workplace aggression can have devastating effects on an organization's employees. For example, it has been found that targets of workplace aggression report lower levels of well-being. Other studies have shown that aggression in the workplace can cause the victims of such behaviors to suffer from health problems. Bjorkqvist, Osterman, and Hjelt-Back even found that targets exhibited symptoms similar to those of post-traumatic stress disorder (PTSD), such as anxiety and depression. Sorensen et al. found possible associations between harassment at work and well-being measures of lower back pain and sleep deficiency among a sample of hospital workers.

Team Performance

Research has looked at the negative impacts of workplace aggression on team performance and particularly team effectiveness as was evidenced in a recent study by Aube and Rousseau.

Job Satisfaction

Victims of workplace aggression may suffer from reduced job satisfaction. Lapierre, Spector, and Leck found that those who perceived being targets of workplace aggression reported significantly lower overall job satisfaction. Similarly, those who perceive abuse from their supervisors report lower levels of job satisfaction.

Gender Differences in Outcomes

Research has shown that males and females react to workplace aggression differently. While both males and females have reported lower well-being after experiencing aggression in the workplace, studies indicate that the relationship between experienced workplace aggression and decreased well-being was stronger for men. In one study, results showed that men who reported more experienced work aggression were more likely to report physical, psychosocial, affective, and cognitive problems. This study also showed that the type of aggression, whether it is overt or covert, did not matter for these outcomes. The study attributes these findings to the idea of modern-day masculinity, which stresses achievement and success in the workplace.

For females, nonsexual aggression has been found to have a stronger impact on job satisfaction than sexual aggression. Also, nonsexual aggression has a stronger relationship with job satisfaction in females than in males.

Prevention

Prevention programs focus on reducing instances of workplace aggression. Programs that incorporate personnel selection, organizational sanctions, and training are recommended.

Personnel Selection

Based on a workplace prevention program developed by the United States Postal Service (USPS), Neuman and Baron encourage organizations to use personnel screening and testing to identify potential employees who are likely to behave aggressively before they are even hired. This proactive strategy prevents individuals who are predisposed to aggress from even entering the workplace.

Organizational Sanctions

Explicit policies regarding workplace aggression may help organizations to reduce aggression. Employees who perceived that their organization would punish workplace aggressors reported less workplace aggression even when their perceptions of interpersonal justice were high. Neuman and Baron also suggest using organizational policies to curb workplace aggression and to shape strong anti-aggressive organizational norms.

Training

Training is also an important part of a prevention program. Neuman and Baron suggest that training for both supervisors and subordinates should focus on teaching employees methods for dealing with aggression. Similarly, Rai advises that appropriate training should inform employees that management takes threats seriously, encourage employees to report incidents, and demonstrate management's commitment to deal with reported incidents.

Organizational Support

Organizational support can influence the effects of workplace aggression. Schat and Kelloway isolated two forms of organizational support: instrumental and informational. Instrumental support refers to providing some type of assistance directly to an afflicted individuals, whereas information support refers to providing employees with self-help informational resources.

Workplace Bullying

Workplace bullying is a persistent pattern of mistreatment from others in the workplace that causes either physical or emotional harm. It can include such tactics as verbal, nonverbal, psychological, physical abuse and humiliation. This type of workplace aggression is particularly difficult because, unlike the typical school bully, workplace bullies often operate within the established rules and policies of their organization and their society. In the majority of cases, bullying in the workplace is reported as having been by someone who has authority over their victim. However, bullies can also be peers, and occasionally subordinates. Research has also investigated the impact of the larger organizational context on bullying as well as the group-level processes that impact on the incidence and maintenance of bullying behaviour. Bullying can be covert or overt. It may be missed by superiors; it may be known by many throughout the organization. Negative effects are not limited to the targeted individuals, and may lead to a decline in employee morale and a change in organizational culture.

First Known Documented use

The first known documented use of "workplace bullying" is in 1992 in a book by Andrea Adams called *Bullying at Work: How to Confront and Overcome It.*

Definitions

While there is no universally accepted formal definition of workplace bullying, several researchers have endeavoured to define it:

- According to Einarsen, Hoel, Zapf and Cooper "Bullying at work means harassing, offending, socially excluding someone or negatively affecting someone's work tasks. In order for the label bullying (or mobbing) to be applied to a particular activity, interaction or process it has to occur repeatedly and regularly (e.g. weekly) and over a period of time (e.g. about six months). Bullying is an escalated process in the course of which the person confronted ends up in an inferior position and becomes the target of systematic negative social acts."

- According to Tracy, Lutgen-Sandvik, and Alberts, researchers associated with the Arizona State University's Project for Wellness and Work-Life, workplace bullying is most often "*a combination of tactics in which numerous types of hostile communication and behaviour are used*"

- Gary and Ruth Namie define workplace bullying as "*repeated, health-harming mistreatment, verbal abuse, or conduct which is threatening, humiliating, intimidating, or sabotage that interferes with work or some combination of the three.*"

- Pamela Lutgen-Sandvik expands this definition, stating that workplace bullying is "*persistent verbal and nonverbal aggression at work, that includes personal attacks, social ostracism, and a multitude of other painful messages and hostile interactions.*"

- Catherine Mattice and Karen Garman define workplace bullying as "*systematic aggressive communication, manipulation of work, and acts aimed at humiliating or degrading one or more individual that create an unhealthy and unprofessional power imbalance between bully and target(s), result in psychological consequences for targets and co-workers, and cost enormous monetary damage to an organization's bottom line*"

- Employers can also be bullies. Bad employers use bullying strategically to rid the workplace of good employees to avoid a legal obligation, such as paying unemployment compensation or a worker's compensation claim. Employers also use bullying tactics to drive out employees who demand legal pay or overtime or assert a legal right to organize collectively. The most common type of complaint filed with the U.S. Equal Employment Opportunity Commission involves retaliation, where an employer harasses or bullies an employee for objecting to illegal discrimination. Patricia Barnes, author of *Surviving Bullies, Queen Bees & Psychopaths in the Workplace*, argues that employers that bully are a critical but often overlooked aspect of the problem in the United States.

Because it can occur in a variety of contexts and forms, it is also useful to define workplace bullying by the key features that these behaviours possess. Bullying is characterized by:

- Repetition (occurs regularly)

- Duration (is enduring)

- Escalation (increasing aggression)

- Power disparity (the target lacks the power to successfully defend themselves).

- Attributed intent

This distinguishes bullying from isolated behaviours and other forms of job stress and allows the term workplace bullying to be applied in various contexts and to behaviours that meet these characteristics. Many observers agree that bullying is often a repetitive behaviour. However, some experts who have dealt with a great many people who report abuse also categorize some once-only events as bullying, for example with cases where there appear to be severe sequelae. Expanding the common understanding of bullying to include single, severe episodes also parallels the legal definitions of sexual harassment in the US.

According to Pamela Lutgin-Sandvik, the lack of unifying language to name the phenomenon of workplace bullying is a problem because without a unifying term or phrase, individuals have difficulty naming their experiences of abuse, and therefore have trouble pursuing justice against the bully. Unlike sexual harassment, which named a specific problem and is now recognized in law of many countries (including U.S.), workplace bullying is still being established as a relevant social problem and is in need of a specific vernacular.

Euphemisms intended to trivialize bullying and its impact on bullied people: incivility, disrespect, difficult people, personality conflict, negative conduct, and ill treatment. Bullied people are labelled as insubordinate when they resist the bullying treatment.

There is no exact definition for bullying behaviours in workplace, which is why different terms and definitions are common. For example, mobbing is a commonly used term in France and Germany, where it refers to a "mob" of bullies, rather than a single bully; this phenomenon is not often seen in other countries. In the United States, aggression and emotional abuse are frequently used terms, whereas harassment is the term preferred in Finland. Workplace bullying is primarily used in Australia, UK, and Northern Europe.

Statistics

Bosses are the most common bullies. In fact, approximately 72% of bullies outrank their victims. Statistics from the 2007 WBI-Zogby survey show that 13% of U.S. employees report being bullied currently, 24% say they have been bullied in the past and an additional 12% say they have witnessed workplace bullying. Nearly half of all American workers (49%) report that they have been affected by workplace bullying, either being a target themselves or having witnessed abusive behaviour against a co-worker.

Although socio-economic factors may play a role in the abuse, researchers from the Project for Wellness and Work-Life suggest that "workplace bullying, by definition, is not explicitly connected to demographic markers such as sex and ethnicity". Because one in ten employees experiences workplace bullying, the prevalence of this issue is cause for great concern, even as initial data about this issue are reviewed.

According to the 2010 National Health Interview Survey Occupational Health Supplement (NHIS-OHS), the national prevalence rate for workers reporting having been threatened, bullied, or harassed by anyone on the job was 8%.

In 2008, Dr. Judy Fisher-Blando wrote a doctoral research dissertation on *Aggressive behaviour: Workplace Bullying and Its Effect on Job Satisfaction and Productivity.* The scientific study determined that almost 75% of employees surveyed had been affected by workplace bullying, whether as a target or a witness. Further research showed the types of bullying behaviour, and organizational support.

Gender

In terms of gender, the Workplace Bullying Institute (2007) states that women appear to be at greater risk of becoming a bullying target, as 57% of those who reported being targeted for abuse were women. Men are more likely to participate in aggressive bullying behaviour (60%), however when the bully is a woman her target is more likely to be a woman as well (71%).

In the research of Samnani and Singh (2012), it concludes the findings from previous 20 years' literature and claims that in terms of the gender factor, inconsistent findings could not support the differences across gender.

The NHIS-OHS confirms the previous finding, as higher prevalence rates for being threatened, bullied, or harassed were identified for women (9%) compared with men (7%).

Race

Race also may play a role in the experience of workplace bullying. According to the Workplace Bullying Institute (2007), the comparison of reported combined bullying (current + ever bullied) prevalence percentages reveals the pattern from most to least:

1. Hispanics (52.1%)
2. Blacks (46%)
3. Whites (33.5%)
4. Asian (30.6%)

The reported rates of witnessing bullying were:

1. Asian (28.5%)
2. Blacks (21.1%)
3. Hispanics (14%)
4. Whites (10.8%)

The percentages of those reporting that they have neither experienced nor witnessed mistreatment were

1. Asians (57.3%)
2. Whites (49.7%)
3. Hispanics (32.2%)
4. Blacks (23.4%)

Research psychologist Tony Buon published one of the first reviews of bullying in China in the prestigious Journal PKU Business Review in 2005.

Marital Status

Higher prevalence rates for experiencing a hostile work environment were identified for divorced or separated workers compared to married workers, widowed workers, and never married workers.

Education

Higher prevalence rates for experiencing a hostile work environment were identified for workers with some college education or workers with high school diploma or GED, compared to workers with less than a high school education.

Age

Lower prevalence rates for experiencing a hostile work environment were identified for workers aged 65 and older compared to workers in other age groups.

With respect to age, conflicting findings have been reported. A study by Einarsen and Skogstad (1996) indicates older employees tend to be more likely to be bullied than younger ones.

Industry

Among industry groups, workers with higher prevalence rates of a hostile work environment, compared to all adults employed at some time in a 12-month period leading up to a survey in 2010 (8%), were in public administration (16%) and retail trade industries (10%). Lower prevalence rates of a hostile work environment were reported among those working in construction (5%); finance and insurance (5%); manufacturing (5%); and professional, scientific, and technical services industries (6%).

Occupation

For occupational groups, workers in protective service reported a higher prevalence rate (25%) of hostile work environments compared to the prevalence rate for all adults employed at some time in the past 12 months. Workers in community and social service occupations also experienced a relatively high rate (16%). Lower prevalence rates were observed among architecture and engineering (4%), computer and mathematical (4%), business and financial operations (5%), and construction and extraction (5%) occupations.

Profiling

Researchers Caitlin Buon and Tony Buon have suggested that attempts to profile 'the bully' have been damaging They state that the "bully" profile is that 'the bully' is always aware of what they are doing, deliberately sets out to harm their 'victims', targets a particular individual or type of person and has some kind of underlying personality flaw, insecurity or disorder. But this is unproven and lacks evidence. The researchers suggest referring to workplace bullying as generic harassment along with other forms of non-specific harassment and this would enable employees to use less emotionally charged language and start a dialogue about their experiences rather than being repelled by the spectre of being labelled as a pathological predator or having to define their experiences as the victims of such a person. Tony Buon and Caitlin Buon also suggest that the perception and profile of the workplace bully is not facilitating interventions with the problem. They suggest that to make significant progress and achieve behaviour change over the long term then organisations and individuals need to embrace the notion that everyone must all potentially house 'the bully' within them and their organisations. It exists in workplace cultures, belief systems, interactions and emotional competencies and cannot be transformed if externalization and demonization continue the problem by profiling 'the bully' rather than talking about behaviours and interpersonal interactions.

Relationship Among Participants

From the research by Hoel, it is clear that most of the perpetrators are supervisors, the second one is peers, subordinates and customers follow which found from Hoel's research. So three main relationships among the participants in workplace bullying can be indicated as:

- between supervisor and subordinate
- among co-workers
- employees and customers
- between organization (organizational institution or system).

Bullying behaviour shows as an abuse of power between supervisors and subordinates in workplace. Supervisors release their own pressure to bully subordinates with their higher power due to workplace bullying. It is always related to management style of the supervisors. An authoritative management style is accompanied by a kind of bullying behaviours which can make subordinates fear so that supervisors can become authority themselves. On the other hand, some researchers agree that bullying behaviours is a positive performance in workplace. Workplace bullying can attribute to the organizational power and control. It is also a representative of power and control. if an organization want to improve this situation in workplace, strategies and policies must be improved. Lacking of policy in bullying like low-monitoring or no punishment will result in tolerating in organization. Bullying behaviours in workplace also exist among colleagues. They can be either the 'target' or perpetrator. If workplace bullying happens among the co-workers, witness will take side between target and perpetrator. Perpetrators always win, because witnesses do not want to be the next target. This way, it does encourage perpetrators to continue this behaviour. In addition, the sense of the injustice by targets might become another perpetrator to bully other colleagues who have less power than them. Varitia who is a workplace bullying researcher investigate that 20% of interviewees who experienced workplace bullying thought the reason why they became a target is they are different from others. In a word, bullying can increase more bullying in workplace. The third relationship in workplace is between employees and customers. Although it takes a little part, it plays a significant role about the efficiency of the organization. If an employee work with unhealthy emotion, it will affect the quality of the service seriously. This relationship is closely related to emotion label. Lots of examples can be listed from our daily life, like customers are ignored by shop assistants, patients are shouted by nurses in the hospital and so on. On the other hand, customers might despise the employees, especially blue-collar job, such as gas station assistants. Bullying behaviours in workplace can generate effect mutually between the employees and customers. The Fourth relationship in workplace is between organization or its institution or its system and the employees. In the article of Andreas Liefooghe (2012), it notes that a lot of employees describe their organization as bully. It is not environmental factors facilitating the bullying but it is the bullying itself. Tremendous power imbalance enables company to "legitimately exercise" their power in the way of monitoring and controlling as bullying. The terms of the bullying "traditionally" imply to interpersonal relationship. Talking about bullying in interpersonal level is legitimate, but talking about the exploitation, justice and subjugation as bullying of organization would be "relatively ridiculous" or not taken as serious. Bullying is sometimes more than purely interpersonal issue.

Organizational Culture

Bullying is seen to be prevalent in organisations where employees and managers feel that they have the support, or at least the implicit blessing, of senior managers to carry on their abusive and bullying behaviour. Furthermore, new managers will quickly come to view this form of behaviour as acceptable and normal if they see others get away with it and are even rewarded for it.

When bullying happens at the highest levels, the effects may be far reaching. That people may be bullied irrespective of their organisational status or rank, including senior managers, indicates the possibility of a negative domino effect, where bullying may be cascaded downwards as the targeted supervisors might offload their own aggression on their subordinates. In such situations, a bullying scenario in the boardroom may actually threaten the productivity of the entire organisation.

Geographical Culture

According to a research investigating the acceptability of the bullying behaviour across from different cultures (Power et al., 2013), it clearly shows that culture could also serve as an influencing factor. The difference on the cultural dimension across different cultures could affect the perception on the acceptable behaviour. National-level factors, such as culture, may also represent a predictor of workplace bullying (Harvey et al., 2009; Hoel et al., 1999; Lutgen-Sandvik et al., 2007).

Humane orientation is negatively associated with the acceptability of bullying for WRB (Work related bullying). Performance orientation is positively associated with the acceptance of bullying. Future orientation is negatively associated with the acceptability of bullying. A culture of femininity suggests that individuals tend to value interpersonal relationships to a greater degree.

Three broad dimensions have been mentioned in relation to workplace bullying: power distance; masculinity versus femininity; and individualism versus collectivism (Lutgen-Sandvik et al., 2007).

In Confucian Asia, which has a higher performance orientation than Latin America and Sub-Saharan Africa, bullying may be seen as an acceptable price to pay for performance. The value Latin America holds for personal connections with employees and the higher humane orientation of Sub-Saharan Africa may help to explain their distaste for bullying. A culture of individualism in the US implies competition, which may increase the likelihood of workplace bullying situations.

Culture of Fear

Ashforth discussed potentially destructive sides of leadership and identified what he referred to as petty tyrants, i.e.Leaders who exercise a tyrannical style of management, resulting in a climate of fear in the workplace. Partial or intermittent negative reinforcement can create an effective climate of fear and doubt. When employees get the sense that bullies “get away with it”, a climate of fear may be the result. Several studies have confirmed a relationship between bullying, on the one hand, and an autocratic leadership and an authoritarian way of settling conflicts or dealing with disagreements, on the other. An authoritarian style of leadership may create a climate of fear, where there is little or no room for dialogue and where complaining may be considered futile.

In a study of public-sector union members, approximately one in five workers reported having considered leaving the workplace as a result of witnessing bullying taking place.

Rayner explained these figures by pointing to the presence of a climate of fear in which employees considered reporting to be unsafe, where bullies had "got away with it" previously despite management knowing of the presence of bullying.

Kiss up Kick Down

The workplace bully is often expert at knowing how to work the system. They can spout all the current management buzzwords about supportive management but basically use it as a cover. By keeping their abusive behaviour hidden, any charges made by individuals about his or her bullying will always come down to your word against his. They may have a *kiss up kick down* personality, wherein they are always highly cooperative, respectful, and caring when talking to upper management but the opposite when it comes to their relationship with those whom they supervise. Bullies tend to ingratiate themselves to their bosses while intimidating subordinates. They may be socially popular with others in management, including those who will determine their fate. Often, a workplace bully will have mastered *kiss up kick down* tactics that hide their abusive side from superiors who review their performance.

As a consequence of this *kiss up kick down* strategy:

- a bully's mistakes are always concealed or blamed on underlings or circumstances beyond their control
- a bully keeps the target under constant stress
- a bully's power base is fear, not respect
- a bully withholds information from subordinates and keeps the information flow top-down only
- a bully blames conflicts and problems on subordinate's lack of competence, poor attitude, and/or character flaws
- a bully creates an unnatural work environment where people constantly walk on eggshells and are compelled to behave in ways they normally would not

Fight or Flight

The most typical reactions to workplace bullying are to do with the survival instinct - "fight or flight" - and these are probably a victim's healthier responses to bullying. Flight is a legitimate and valid response to bullying. It is very common, especially in organizations in which upper management cannot or will not deal with the bullying. In hard economic times, however, flight may not be an option, and fighting may be the only choice.

Fighting the bullying can require near heroic action, especially if the bullying targets just one or two individuals. It can also be a difficult challenge. There are some times when confrontation is called for. First, there is always a chance that the bully boss is labouring under the impression that this is the way to get things done and does not recognize the havoc being wreaked on subordinates.

Typology of Bullying Behaviours

With some variations, the following typology of workplace bullying behaviours has been adopted by a number of academic researchers. The typology uses five different categories.

1. Threat to professional status – including belittling opinions, public professional humiliation, accusations regarding lack of effort, intimidating use of discipline or competence procedures
2. Threat to personal standing – including undermining personal integrity, destructive innuendo and sarcasm, making inappropriate jokes about target, persistent teasing, name calling, insults, intimidation
3. Isolation – including preventing access to opportunities, physical or social isolation, withholding necessary information, keeping the target out of the loop, ignoring or excluding
4. Overwork – including undue pressure, impossible deadlines, unnecessary disruptions.
5. Destabilisation – including failure to acknowledge good work, allocation of meaningless tasks, removal of responsibility, repeated reminders of blunders, setting target up to fail, shifting goal posts without telling the target.

Tactics

Research by the Workplace Bullying Institute, suggests that the following are the 25 most common workplace bullying tactics:

1. Falsely accused someone of "errors" not actually made (71 percent).
2. Stared, glared, was nonverbally intimidating and was clearly showing hostility (68 percent).
3. Unjustly discounted the person's thoughts or feelings ("oh, that's silly") in meetings (64 percent).
4. Used the "silent treatment" to "ice out" and separate from others (64 percent).
5. Exhibited presumably uncontrollable mood swings in front of the group (61 percent).
6. Made-up rules on the fly that even she/he did not follow (61 percent).

7. Disregarded satisfactory or exemplary quality of completed work despite evidence (discrediting) (58 percent).
8. Harshly and constantly criticized having a different standard for the target (57 percent).
9. Started, or failed to stop, destructive rumours or gossip about the person (56 percent).
10. Encouraged people to turn against the person being tormented (55 percent).
11. Singled out and isolated one person from other co-workers, either socially or physically (54 percent).
12. Publicly displayed gross, undignified, but not illegal, behaviour (53 percent).
13. Yelled, screamed, threw tantrums in front of others to humiliate a person (53 percent).
14. Stole credit for work done by others (plagiarism) (47 percent).
15. Abused the evaluation process by lying about the person's performance (46 percent).
16. Declared target "insubordinate" for failing to follow arbitrary commands (46 percent).
17. Used confidential information about a person to humiliate privately or publicly (45 percent).
18. Retaliated against the person after a complaint was filed (45 percent).
19. Made verbal put-downs/insults based on gender, race, accent, age or language, disability (44 percent).
20. Assigned undesirable work as punishment (44 percent).
21. Created unrealistic demands (workload, deadlines, duties) for person singled out (44 percent).
22. Launched a baseless campaign to oust the person; effort not stopped by the employer (43 percent).
23. Encouraged the person to quit or transfer rather than to face more mistreatment (43 percent).
24. Sabotaged the person's contribution to a team goal and reward (41 percent).
25. Ensured failure of person's project by not performing required tasks, such as sign-offs, taking calls, working with collaborators (40 percent)

Abusive Workplace Behaviours

According to Bassman, common abusive workplace behaviours are:

1. Disrespecting and devaluing the individual, often through disrespectful and devaluing language or verbal abuse
2. Overwork and devaluation of personal life (particularly salaried workers who are not compensated)
3. Harassment through micromanagement of tasks and time
4. Over evaluation and manipulating information (for example concentration on negative characteristics and failures, setting up subordinate for failure).
5. Managing by threat and intimidation
6. Stealing credit and taking unfair advantage
7. Preventing access to opportunities
8. Downgrading an employee's capabilities to justify downsizing
9. Impulsive destructive behaviour

According to Hoel and Cooper, common abusive workplace behaviours are:

1. Having opinions and views ignored
2. Withholding information which affects the target's performance
3. Being exposed to an unmanageable workload
4. Being given tasks with unreasonable or impossible targets or deadlines
5. Being ordered to do work below competence
6. Being ignored or facing hostility when the target approaches
7. Being humiliated or ridiculed in connection with work
8. Excessive monitoring of a person's work
9. Spreading gossip
10. Insulting or offensive remarks made about the target's person (i.e. habits and background), attitudes or private life
11. Having key areas of responsibility removed or replaced with more trivial or unpleasant tasks.

Abusive cyberbullying in the workplace can have serious socioeconomic and psychological consequences on the victim. Workplace cyberbullying can lead to sick leave due to depression which in turn can lead to loss of profits for the organisation.

In Specific Professions

Academia

Several aspects of academia, such as the generally decentralized nature of academic institutions and the particular recruitment and career procedures, lend themselves to the practice of bullying and discourage its reporting and mitigation.

Blue-collar Jobs

Bullying has been identified as prominent in blue collar jobs including on the oil rigs and in mechanic shops and machine shops. It is thought that intimidation and fear of retribution cause decreased incident reports. This is also an industry dominated by males, where disclosure of incidents are seen as effeminate, which, in the socioeconomic and cultural milieu of such industries, would likely lead to a vicious circle. This is often used in combination with manipulation and coercion of facts to gain favour among higher ranking administrators.

Information Technology

A culture of bullying is common in information technology (IT), leading to high sickness rates, low morale, poor productivity and high staff turnover. Deadline-driven project work and stressed-out managers take their toll on IT workers.

Medicine

Bullying in the medical profession is common, particularly of student or trainee doctors. It is thought that this is at least in part an outcome of conservative traditional hierarchical structures and teaching methods in the medical profession which may result in a bullying cycle.

Nursing

Bullying has been identified as being particularly prevalent in the nursing profession although the reasons are not clear. It is thought that relational aggression (psychological aspects of bullying such as gossiping and intimidation) are relevant. Relational aggression has been studied amongst girls but not so much amongst adult women.

Teaching

School teachers are commonly the subject of bullying but they are also sometimes the originators of bullying within a school environment.

Legal Profession

Bullying in the legal profession is believed to be more common than in some other professions. It is believed that its adversarial, hierarchical tradition contributes towards this. Women, trainees and solicitors who have been qualified for five years or less are more impacted, as are ethnic minority lawyers and lesbian, gay and bisexual lawyers.

Military

Bullying exists to varying degrees in the military of some countries, often involving various forms of hazing or abuse by higher members of the military hierarchy.

Forms

Tim Field suggested that workplace bullying takes these forms:

- Serial bullying — the source of all dysfunction can be traced to one individual, who picks on one employee after another and destroys them, then moves on. Probably the most common type of bullying.
- Secondary bullying — the pressure of having to deal with a serial bully causes the general behaviour to decline and sink to the lowest level.
- Pair bullying — this takes place with two people, one active and verbal, the other often watching and listening.
- Gang bullying or group bullying — is a serial bully with colleagues. Gangs can occur anywhere, but flourish in corporate bullying climates. It is often called mobbing and usually involves scapegoating and victimisation.
- Vicarious bullying — two parties are encouraged to fight. This is the typical "triangulation" where the aggression gets passed around.
- Regulation bullying — where a serial bully forces their target to comply with rules, regulations, procedures or laws regardless of their appropriateness, applicability or necessity.
- Residual bullying — after the serial bully has left or been fired, the behaviour continues. It can go on for years.
- Legal bullying — the bringing of a vexatious legal action to control and punish a person.
- Pressure bullying or unwitting bullying — having to work to unrealistic time scales and/or inadequate resources.
- Corporate bullying — where an employer abuses an employee with impunity, knowing the law is weak and the job market is soft.

- Organizational bullying – a combination of pressure bullying and corporate bullying. Occurs when an organization struggles to adapt to changing markets, reduced income, cuts in budgets, imposed expectations and other extreme pressures.
- Institutional bullying – entrenched and is accepted as part of the culture.
- Client bullying – an employee is bullied by those they serve, for instance subway attendants or public servants.
- Cyber bullying – the use of information and communication technologies to support deliberate, repeated, and hostile behaviour by an individual or group, that is intended to harm others.

Adult bullying can come in an assortment of forms. There are about five distinctive types of adult bullies. A narcissistic bully is described as a self-centred person whose egotism is frail and possesses the need to put others down. An impulsive bully is someone who acts on bullying based on stress or being upset at the moment. A physical bully uses physical injury and the threat of harm to abuse their victims, while a verbal bully uses demeaning and cynicism to debase their victims. Lastly, a secondary adult bully is portrayed as a person that did not start the initial bullying but participates in afterwards to avoid being bullied themselves ("Adult Bullying").

Emotional Intelligence

Workplace bullying is reported to be far more prevalent than perhaps commonly thought. For some reason, workplace bullying seems to be particularly widespread in healthcare organizations; 80% of nurses report experiencing workplace bullying. Similar to the school environment for children, the work environment typically places groups of adult peers together in a shared space on a regular basis. In such a situation, social interactions and relationships are of great importance to the function of the organizational structure and in pursuing goals. The emotional consequences of bullying put an organization at risk of losing victimized employees. Bullying also contributes to a negative work environment, is not conducive to necessary cooperation and can lessen productivity at various levels. Bullying in the workplace is associated with negative responses to stress. The ability to manage emotions, especially emotional stress, seems to be a consistently important factor in different types of bullying. The workplace in general can be a stressful environment, so a negative way of coping with stress or an inability to do so can be particularly damning. Workplace bullies may have high social intelligence and low emotional intelligence (EI). In this context, bullies tend to rank high on the social ladder and are adept at influencing others. The combination of high social intelligence and low empathy is conducive to manipulative behaviour, such that Hutchinson (2013) describes workplace bullying to be. In working groups where employees have low EI, workers can be persuaded to engage in unethical behaviour. With the bullies' persuasion, the work group is socialized in a way that rationalizes the behaviour, and makes the group tolerant or supportive of the bullying. Hutchinson & Hurley (2013) make the case that EI and leadership skills are both necessary to bullying intervention in the workplace, and illustrates the relationship between EI, leadership and reductions in bullying. EI and ethical behaviour among other members of the work team have been shown to have a significant impact on ethical behaviour of nursing teams. Higher EI is linked to improvements in the work environment and is an important moderator between conflict and reactions to conflict in the workplace. The self-awareness and self-management dimensions of EI have both been illustrated to have strong positive correlations with effective leadership and the specific leadership ability to build healthy work environments and work culture.

Related Concepts

Abusive Supervision

Abusive supervision overlaps with workplace bullying in the workplace context. Research suggests that 75% of workplace bullying incidents are perpetrated by hierarchically superior agents. Abusive supervision differs from related constructs such as supervisor bullying and undermining in that it does not describe the intentions or objectives of the supervisor.

Power and Control

A power and control model has been developed for the workplace, divided into the following categories:

- overt actions
- covert actions
- emotional control
- isolation
- economic control
- tactics
- restrictions
- management privilege.

Workplace Mobbing

Workplace mobbing overlaps with workplace bullying. The concept originated from the study of animal behaviour. It concentrates on bullying by a group.

Workplace Incivility

Workplace bullying overlaps to some degree with workplace incivility but tends to encompass more intense and typically repeated acts of disregard and rudeness. Negative spirals of increasing incivility between organizational members can result in bullying, but isolated acts of incivility are not conceptually bullying despite the apparent similarity in their form and content. In case of bullying, the intent of harm is less ambiguous, an unequal balance of power (both formal and informal) is more salient, and the target of bullying feels threatened, vulnerable and unable to defend himself or herself against negative recurring actions.

Personality Disorders and Dysfunctional Personality Characteristics

Executives

In 2005, psychologists Belinda Board and Katarina Fritzon at the University of Surrey, UK, interviewed and gave personality tests to high-level British executives and compared their profiles with those of criminal psychiatric patients at Broadmoor Hospital in the UK. They found that three out of eleven personality disorders were actually more common in executives than in the disturbed criminals. They were:

- Histrionic personality disorder: including superficial charm, insincerity, egocentricity and manipulation
- Narcissistic personality disorder: including grandiosity, self-focused lack of empathy for others, exploitativeness and independence.
- Obsessive-compulsive personality disorder: including perfectionism, excessive devotion to work, rigidity, stubbornness and dictatorial tendencies.

They described these business people as successful psychopaths and the criminals as unsuccessful psychopaths.

According to leading leadership academic Manfred F.R. Kets de Vries, it seems almost inevitable these days that there will be some personality disorders in a senior management team.

Industrial/organizational psychology research has also examined the types of bullying that exist among business professionals and the prevalence of this form of bullying in the workplace as well as ways to measure bullying empirically.

Psychopathy

Narcissism, lack of self-regulation, lack of remorse and lack of conscience have been identified as traits displayed by bullies. These traits are shared with psychopaths, indicating that there is some theoretical cross-over between bullies and psychopaths. Bullying is used by corporate psychopaths as a tactic to humiliate subordinates. Bullying is also used as a tactic to scare, confuse and disorient those who may be a threat to the activities of the corporate psychopath Using meta data analysis on hundreds of UK research papers, Boddy concluded that 36% of bullying incidents were caused by the presence of corporate psychopaths. According to Boddy there are two types of bullying:

- predatory bullying - the bully just enjoys bullying and tormenting vulnerable people for the sake of it
- instrumental bullying - the bullying is for a purpose, helping the bully achieve his goals.

A corporate psychopath uses instrumental bullying to further his goals of promotion and power as the result of causing confusion and divide and rule.

People with high scores on a psychopathy rating scale are more likely to engage in bullying, crime and drug use than other people. Hare and Babiak noted that about 29 per cent of corporate psychopaths are also bullies. Other research has also shown that people with high scores on a psychopathy rating scale were more likely to engage in bullying, again indicating that psychopaths tend to be bullies in the workplace.

A workplace bully or abuser will often have issues with social functioning. These types of people often have psychopathic traits that are difficult to identify in the hiring and promotion process. These individuals often lack anger management skills and have a distorted sense of reality. Consequently, when confronted with the accusation of abuse, the abuser is not aware that any harm was done.

Narcissism

In 2007, researchers Catherine Mattice and Brian Spitzberg at San Diego State University, USA, found that narcissism revealed a positive relationship with bullying. Narcissists were found to prefer indirect bullying tactics (such as withholding information that affects others' performance, ignoring others, spreading gossip, constantly reminding others of mistakes, ordering others to do work below their competence level, and excessively monitoring others' work) rather than direct tactics (such as making threats, shouting, persistently criticizing, or making false allegations). The research also revealed that narcissists are highly motivated to bully, and that to some extent, they are left with feelings of satisfaction after a bullying incident occurs.

Machiavellianism

According to Namie, Machiavellians manipulate and exploit others to advance their perceived personal agendas but he emphasizes that they are not mentally ill. They do not have a personality disorder, schizophrenia and neither are they psychopaths. In his view, Machiavellianism represents the core of workplace bullying.

Health Effects

According to Gary and Ruth Namie, as well as Tracy, et al., workplace bullying can harm the health of the targets of bullying. Organizations are beginning to take note of workplace bullying because of the costs to the organization in terms of the health of their employees.

According to scholars at The Project for Wellness and Work-Life at Arizona State University, "workplace bullying is linked to a host of physical, psychological, organizational, and social costs." Stress is the most predominant health effect associated with bullying in the workplace. Research indicates that workplace stress has significant negative effects that are correlated to poor mental health and poor physical health, resulting in an increase in the use of "sick days" or time off from work (Farrell & Geist-Martin, 2005).

The negative effects of bullying are so severe that posttraumatic stress disorder (PTSD) and even suicide are not uncommon. Tehrani found that 1 in 10 targets experience PTSD, and that 44% of her respondents experienced PTSD similar to that of battered women and victims of child abuse. Matthiesen and Einarsen found that up to 77% of targets experience PTSD.

In addition, co-workers who witness workplace bullying can also have negative effects, such as fear, stress, and emotional exhaustion. Those who witness repetitive workplace abuse often choose to leave the place of employment where the abuse took place. Workplace bullying can also hinder the organizational dynamics such as group cohesion, peer communication, and overall performance.

According to the 2012 survey conducted by Workplace Bullying Institute (516 respondents), Anticipation of next negative event is the most common psychological symptom of workplace bullying reported by 80%. Panic attacks afflict 52%. Half (49%) of targets reported being diagnosed with clinical depression. Sleep disruption, loss of concentration, mood swings, and pervasive sadness and insomnia were more common (ranging from 77% to 50%). Nearly three-quarters (71%) of targets sought treatment from a physician. Over half (63%) saw a mental health professional for their work-related symptoms. Respondents reported other symptoms that can be exacerbated by stress: migraine headaches (48%), irritable bowel disorder (37%), chronic fatigue syndrome (33%) and sexual dysfunction (27%).

Financial costs to Employers

Several studies have attempted to quantify the cost of bullying to an organization.

- According to the National Institute of Occupational Safety Health (NIOSH) mental illness among the workforce leads to a loss in employment amounting to $19 billion and a drop in productivity of $3 billion (Sauter, et al., 1990).

- In a report commissioned by the ILO, Hoel, Sparks, & Cooper did a comprehensive analysis of the costs involved in bullying. They estimated a cost 1.88 Billion Pounds plus the cost of lost productivity.
- Based on replacement cost of those who leave as a result of being bullied or witnessing bullying, Rayner and Keashly (2004) estimated that for an organization of 1,000 people, the cost would be $1.2 million US. This estimate did not include the cost of litigation should victims bring suit against the organization.
- A recent Finnish study of more than 5,000 hospital staff found that those who had been bullied had 26% more certified sickness absence than those who were not bullied, when figures were adjusted for base-line measures one year prior to the survey (Kivimaki et al., 2000). According to the researchers these figures are probably an underestimation as many of the targets are likely to have been bullied already at the time the base-line measures were obtained.

Research by Dr. Dan Dana has shown organizations suffer a large financial cost by not accurately managing conflict and bullying type behaviours. He has developed a tool to assist with calculating the cost of conflict. In addition, researcher Tamara Parris discusses how employers need to be more attentive in managing various discordant behaviours in the workplace, such as, bullying, as it not only creates a financial cost to the organization, but also erodes the company's human resources assets.

References

- McIvor, A.J. (1987), "Employers, the government, and industrial fatigue in Britain, 1890-1918", British Journal of Industrial Medicine, 44: 724–732, doi:10.1136/oem.44.11.724
- Ludy T. Benjamin (2007), "Lillian Gilbreth's Engineering Psychology", A brief history of modern psychology, Wiley-Blackwell, p. 105, ISBN 978-1-4051-3205-3
- Stanton, N. (1996). "Engineering Psychology: Another Science of Common Sense?". The Psychologist. 9 (7): 300–303. Retrieved 2 July 2011
- Kong, Y. K.; Lowe, B. D.; Lee, S. J.; Krieg, E. F. (2007). "Evaluation of handle design characteristics in a maximum screwdriving torque task". Ergonomics. 50 (9): 1404–1418. doi:10.1080/00140130701393775
- Rai, S. (2002). "Preventing workplace aggression and violence—A role for occupational therapy". Journal of Prevention, Assessment, and Rehabilitation. 18 (15–22): 15–22. PMID 12441587
- Schultz, Duane P. Schultz, Sydney Ellen (2010). Psychology and work today : an introduction to industrial and organizational psychology (10th ed.). Upper Saddle River, N.J.: Prentice Hall. p. 384. ISBN 978-0205683581
- Williams, Ray (3 May 2011). "The Silent Epidemic: Workplace Bullying". Psychology Today. Archived from the original on 2016-06-11. Retrieved 2016-11-13

- Braiker, Harriet B. (2004). Who's Pulling Your Strings ? How to Break The Cycle of Manipulation. ISBN 0-07-144672-9
- "Project for Wellness and Work-Life (PWWL) | Human Communication". Humancommunication.clas.asu.edu. Archived from the original on 10 December 2012. Retrieved 2013-04-18
- Harvey, S.; Keashly, L. (2003). "Predicting the risk for aggression in the workplace: Risk factors, self-esteem, and time at work". Social Behavior and Personality. 31: 807–814. doi:10.2224/sbp.2003.31.8.807
- MAARIT VARTIA, 1996. The sources of bullying–psychological work environment and organizational climate. European Journal of Work and Organizational Psychology, 5(2), pp. 203-214
- C. K. Gunsalus (30 September 2006). The college administrator's survival guide. Harvard University Press. pp. 124–125. ISBN 978-0-674-02315-4. Retrieved 7 March 2011
- "Mattice, C.M., & Garman, K. (June 2010). Proactive Solutions for Workplace Bullying: Looking at the Benefits of Positive Psychology.". Retrieved 2013-04-18
- Salin, D. (2001). Prevalence and forms of bullying among business professionals: A comparison of two different strategies for measuring bullying. European Journal of Work and Organizational Psychology, 10, 425-441
- Robert Cantwell; Jill Scevak (August 2009). An Academic Life: A Handbook for New Academics. Australian Council for Educational Research. p. 168. ISBN 978-0-86431-908-1. Retrieved 8 March 2011
- "Workplace Bullying Institute Top 25 workplace bullying tactics". Workplacebullying.org. 29 April 2011. Archived from the original on 2016-08-18. Retrieved 2015-03-26
- Driscoll, R.; Worthington, K.; Hurrell, J.J. (1995). "Workplace assault: An emerging job stressor". Consult Psychological Practical Research. 47: 205–211. doi:10.1037/1061-4087.47.4.205
- Matthiesen, S.B., & Einarsen, S. (2004). Psychiatric distress and symptoms of PTSD among victims of bullying at work. British Journal of Guidance & Counselling, 32, 335–356
- Notelaers, Guy. "Exploring Risk Groups and Risk Factors for Workplace Bullying (Guy Notelaers) - Academia.edu". Unimaas.academia.edu. Retrieved 2012-03-20

Permissions

All chapters in this book are published with permission under the Creative Commons Attribution Share Alike License or equivalent. Every chapter published in this book has been scrutinized by our experts. Their significance has been extensively debated. The topics covered herein carry significant information for a comprehensive understanding. They may even be implemented as practical applications or may be referred to as a beginning point for further studies.

We would like to thank the editorial team for lending their expertise to make the book truly unique. They have played a crucial role in the development of this book. Without their invaluable contributions this book wouldn't have been possible. They have made vital efforts to compile up to date information on the varied aspects of this subject to make this book a valuable addition to the collection of many professionals and students.

This book was conceptualized with the vision of imparting up-to-date and integrated information in this field. To ensure the same, a matchless editorial board was set up. Every individual on the board went through rigorous rounds of assessment to prove their worth. After which they invested a large part of their time researching and compiling the most relevant data for our readers.

The editorial board has been involved in producing this book since its inception. They have spent rigorous hours researching and exploring the diverse topics which have resulted in the successful publishing of this book. They have passed on their knowledge of decades through this book. To expedite this challenging task, the publisher supported the team at every step. A small team of assistant editors was also appointed to further simplify the editing procedure and attain best results for the readers.

Apart from the editorial board, the designing team has also invested a significant amount of their time in understanding the subject and creating the most relevant covers. They scrutinized every image to scout for the most suitable representation of the subject and create an appropriate cover for the book.

The publishing team has been an ardent support to the editorial, designing and production team. Their endless efforts to recruit the best for this project, has resulted in the accomplishment of this book. They are a veteran in the field of academics and their pool of knowledge is as vast as their experience in printing. Their expertise and guidance has proved useful at every step. Their uncompromising quality standards have made this book an exceptional effort. Their encouragement from time to time has been an inspiration for everyone.

The publisher and the editorial board hope that this book will prove to be a valuable piece of knowledge for students, practitioners and scholars across the globe.

Index